The
# THYROID
# HORMONE
Breakthrough

# The
# THYROID
# HORMONE
# Breakthrough

*Overcoming Sexual and*
*Hormonal Problems at Every Age*

## Mary J. Shomon

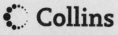

**Collins**
*An Imprint of HarperCollinsPublishers*

*For my husband Jon, the loving, funny, and always*

*patient guy holding my hand and riding right alongside*

*me on my hormonal roller coaster*

THE THYROID HORMONE BREAKTHROUGH. Copyright © 2006 by Mary J. Shomon. All rights reserved. Printed in the United States of America. No part of this book may be used or reproduced in any manner whatsoever without written permission except in the case of brief quotations embodied in critical articles and reviews. For information, address HarperCollins Publishers Inc., 10 East 53rd Street, New York, NY 10022.

HarperCollins books may be purchased for educational, business, or sales promotional use. For information, please write: Special Markets Department, HarperCollins Publishers Inc., 10 East 53rd Street, New York, NY 10022.

FIRST EDITION

Designed by Nicola Ferguson

Library of Congress Cataloging-in-Publication Data has been applied for.

ISBN-13: 978-0-06-079865-9

ISBN-10: 0-06-079865-3

03  04  05  06  07  [APX/RRD]  10  9  8  7  6  5  4  3  2  1

We are volcanoes. When we women offer our experience as our truth, as human truth, all the maps change. There are new mountains.
—*Ursula K. Le Guin*

A small group of thoughtful people can change the world. Indeed it is the only thing that ever has.
—*Margaret Mead*

# ACKNOWLEDGMENTS

On the home front, thanks for my family—Jon, Julia, and Danny—who are so supportive and patient and quick with the hugs and kisses as I get deep into a book project. And my sister/friend Jeannie Yamine—thanks for always being ready to listen, brainstorm, and cheer me on.

I'm also thankful for the love and support of the rest of the family: my father, Dan Shomon; my brother, Dan Shomon Jr.; my in-laws Rus and Barb Mathis; and the family booster club—my aunt, Rita Kelleher, and my cousins, Ellen Blaze and Joan Kelleher. And I never forget my mom, Patricia Rita Shomon, who is always with me.

On the writing front, Sarah Durand of HarperCollins always knows what will make a good book, and she makes my books smarter and better. I'm thrilled she's my editor, aided by the terrific Jeremy Cesarec. And I am grateful for the help and support of Carol Mann, the agent a writer dreams of. I'm so lucky, because my dreams came true!

Thanks to the doctors who keep challenging the norms and breaking new ground, especially my good friends Richard and Karilee Shames and Jacob Teitelbaum. I am also grateful to these medical practitioners for their valuable contributions to this book: Dr. Ken Blanchard, Dr. Michael Borkin,

Dr. David Brownstein, Dr. Ted Friedman, Dr. Steven Hotze, Dr. Steven Langer, Dr. Viana Muller, and Dr. Sherrill Sellman.

Thanks to Hadley Sharp for her excellent work on the Resources section, and to Beth Moeller, Michelle Bahumian, and Caitlyn Conley, whose contributions to keeping the whole thyroid "enterprise" and website going have allowed me to focus on the book. And I cannot forget the unofficial health news bureau—Kim Carmichael Cox, Sherry Leu, and Dottye Howard—who are generous with their time and make sure I don't miss valuable information, news, links, and announcements. Special thanks to the indefatigable Julia Schopick, who is always an inspiration!

I thank the friends who bring joy, inspiration, laughter, good conversation—and often good wine—to my life. Thanks to Mohammed Antabli and Franca Fiabane, Faris Bouhafa and Abla Majaj, Ric and Diane Blake, Michael Phillips and Samantha Shub, Wendy Sobey and Jim Strick, Nadia Krupnikova and Mark Silinsky, Gen Piturro and Demo DeMartile, Jane and Joe Frank, Cynthia and David Austin, Laura Horton, and Kim Conley.

Thanks to the About.com crew—my editor, Dave Johns, who is a great pleasure to work with, and my fellow guides, who are smart, interesting, committed writers, researchers, and advocates who provide such tremendous input and support. In particular, thanks to Phylameana lila Desy of Healing.about.com, Dr. Rich Fogoros of Heartdisease.about.com, and Dr. Vince Ianelli of Pediatrics.about.com. And of course, many thanks to my comrade in "living well," Teri Robert, of Headaches.about.com and author of *Living Well with Migraine Disease and Headaches*.

Finally, I owe my health to the doctors and experts who keep me going personally, including Dr. Kate Lemmerman of the Kaplan Clinic in Arlington, Virginia; my osteopath, Dr. Scott Kwiatkowski of Bethesda, Maryland; my personal trainer, Silvia Treves; and Dr. Jan Nicholson.

May you all live well!

# CONTENTS

# INTRODUCTION

As women, we've come to expect that certain things are inevitable. As young girls, we anticipate—but at the same time dread—the first arrival of "Aunt Flo" or "my friend." Then, for the next 30 to 40 years, we assume that premenstrual syndrome, erratic cycles, and unusually light or heavy menstrual periods are simply an unavoidable part of life.

In the meantime, women's magazines and television news programs deliver conflicting messages: you can get pregnant from a single sexual encounter, but infertility is on the rise. Teenage pregnancy rates are down, but if you're a 45-year-old celebrity, it's a breeze to give birth to twins. If you can't get pregnant after trying for a year, your doctor says you are "experiencing infertility" and shuttles you off to a fertility expert for elaborate and expensive workups. After that you're offered costly procedures and treatments—everything from hormone treatments to in vitro fertilization—to help you have a baby.

When we are pregnant, we assume that morning sickness is to be expected—even the kind of morning sickness that goes on all day and all night throughout the pregnancy, leaving us dehydrated and debilitated. "Morning sickness is a good sign," say the old wives' tales, and our mothers, relatives, and friends repeat this mantra, while prescribing crackers and club soda, as if that will make it better.

And while we all want to be like the celebrity model who still has an adorable figure with a tiny baby "bump" when she's nine months pregnant, and who gets back into size 4 jeans a few weeks later, baby at her breast, some of us definitely don't fit into that category. Instead, we walk around feeling down in the dumps, because our hair is falling out and we have no energy. And we have a horrible feeling of guilt and failure, because we're not making enough milk to breastfeed our baby properly. We need to supplement with formula, or worse—we can't nurse at all.

Many of us just assume that we're not going to have the sex drive that we had when we were young. After reading all those women's magazines and watching enough Oprah and Discovery Channel health shows, who of us can't recite the reasons for our low libido? Marriage, exhaustion, children, not enough time, stress—I could go on for pages listing all the reasons why "losing that spark" is an expected part of life for women.

Let's not forget the hormonal grand finale: menopause. Now that hormone replacement therapy is in the medical doghouse, women are once again saddled with weight gain, hot flashes, night sweats, fatigue, mood swings, vaginal dryness, and low sex drive. And just to add to the fun, we now have something called *perimenopause*—the time before true menopause, when we have all those so-called menopausal symptoms, *plus* erratic and sometimes extremely heavy periods. It may come as a surprise to you—it sure did to me—that perimenopause can go on for as long as a decade!

Have I depressed you yet? You were already depressed, you say? And sort of stressed out and anxious too? Of course, depression and anxiety are conditions that we assume are a given in today's modern life. Antidepressants and antianxiety drugs like Zoloft, Prozac, Effexor, and Zyprexa are among the most prescribed medicines in the United States today.

It may sound as if we women are destined to be victims of our hormones from our preteens into our golden years. But there is hope. And it comes from your thyroid—a small gland that is very powerful, but often overlooked when it comes to women's complaints.

The thyroid is a bowtie- or butterfly-shaped gland located in the neck, below and behind the Adam's apple area. It is the master gland of energy and metabolism, and a key player in our complex endocrine system, interacting with other endocrine glands such as the pancreas, adrenals, ovaries, and pituitary. The thyroid releases hormones that rise and fall in concert with other endocrine hormones, such as insulin, cortisol, estrogen, and testosterone.

When the thyroid is not doing its job properly, it can throw the body's entire hormonal and reproductive systems out of balance.

An undiagnosed or improperly treated thyroid condition may actually be at the root of many symptoms and complaints that we assume are simply "hormonal."

By conservative standards, there are almost 27 million people with thyroid conditions in the United States today. An estimated half of these people are undiagnosed.

And this estimate may just be the tip of the iceberg. Since 2002, experts in the endocrinology community have been calling for changes in the standards that define normal thyroid function. Some doctors are already using new standards for diagnosis and treatment, but many practitioners have yet to adopt them. According to these new standards approximately 59 million Americans are considered to have thyroid disease.

This means that, right now, according to the newly recommended standards, there are as many as 30 million Americans who don't even know they have a thyroid problem. Millions more have been diagnosed and treated, but they may still struggle with related symptoms and side effects. And since thyroid disease affects women seven times more often than men, the vast majority of the undiagnosed are women.

You may have in your mind what many consider the stereotypical thyroid patient...a middle-aged, overweight woman. And if that's not you, you might assume you can't have a thyroid condition. Or you may think that only if you have an enlarged thyroid, known as a goiter, or bulging eyes could you have a thyroid problem. You may have even been told by a doctor, as one young mother was, "You can't possibly have a thyroid problem, because if you did, you wouldn't have been able to just have a baby!"

But being of normal weight, having a normal neck or eyes, or the fact that you were able to have a baby do not rule out a thyroid problem.

That's why I've written this book. In *The Thyroid Hormone Breakthrough*, you'll learn about the thyroid's powerful connection to so many seemingly unrelated hormonal symptoms and complaints, and why this important gland is so often overlooked. You'll learn about the common risk factors for thyroid disease and the symptoms that can help you pinpoint a condition. You'll learn about how to get a proper diagnosis and how treatment can improve your condition. And you'll learn about additional treatments, both conventional and alternative, that can help you enjoy a lifetime of better health.

This book is for you if are experiencing any of these problems:

- You suffer with erratic menstrual periods that may be very heavy or very light, with cycles as short as every 18 days or as long as every 60 days, lasting anywhere from 2 to 10 days. From your first period as an adolescent to the final period that signals the onset of menopause, thyroid imbalances can cause a whole array of menstrual difficulties, including irregular cycles and severe PMS.

- You're unable to get pregnant, or you've had several miscarriages. You may even have undergone expensive and invasive procedures to overcome these problems. An undiagnosed thyroid problem may be the real reason you can't get pregnant.

- You're pregnant, and gaining—or losing—a great deal of weight, perhaps even suffering from severe morning sickness or other debilitating symptoms. Undiagnosed or improperly treated thyroid conditions can worsen your pregnancy symptoms, and even endanger your pregnancy, increasing the risk of miscarriage, intrauterine growth retardation, preterm labor, stillbirth, and cognitive problems or mental retardation in your child.

- You're having a difficult time breastfeeding and losing the baby weight, and you're feeling fatigued, losing your hair, and suffering from postpartum blues. The postpartum period is a common time for thyroid symptoms to appear. And undiagnosed or undertreated postpartum thyroid problems are a key factor behind low milk supply.

- You have little or no interest in sex. We may think this is just the way it is after being married a few years, having children, or getting older, but libido is closely linked to thyroid function. What you think is just low libido may actually be a symptom of a dysfunctional thyroid.

- You're in your forties or fifties, and you are having a particularly difficult perimenopause or severe menopause symptoms. Many women assume that symptoms such as fatigue, weight gain, hair loss, anxiety, and depression are "normal" for women approaching or going through menopause. But in reality, this is also a common time for thyroid problems to appear, and the symptoms being attributed to menopause may actually be caused by a treatable thyroid condition.

Before I continue, I'd like to explain my own background. I'm not a doctor or health professional. I have a degree in international studies from Georgetown University. I never expected to be writing books about thyroid disease. But back in 1995, at the age of 33, I was diagnosed with Hashimoto's disease, an autoimmune condition that causes hypothyroidism. The diagnosis was a turning point in my life and in my career. First, I struggled to return to good health myself. Later, I expanded my own research, began to share this knowledge with others, and became a patient advocate. In 1997, I started a popular, patient-oriented website on thyroid disease, www.thyroid-info.com. In 1998, I launched the only independent print and e-mail newsletter on thyroid health and treatment from a conventional and alternative perspective. I've also written a number of books and magazine articles to help people overcome their health challenges.

Now I get hundreds of e-mails and letters each week from readers all over the world sharing their stories and looking for solutions to their own thyroid and hormonal problems. And I can relate. When it comes to hormonal ups and downs, I've had a few of my own.

I've gone through phases where my periods have been wildly unpredictable, sometimes coming every 21 days, and other times, every 37 days.

In 1997, when I was 35, my husband and I began trying to conceive a child—but only after I had a thorough understanding of my fertility cycles and had my thyroid condition under control and carefully monitored. Thanks to this extra planning, preparation, and knowledge, our daughter was conceived fairly quickly, and was born a happy and healthy 8½ pounds in late 1997. (Don't let anyone tell you that a thyroid problem means you *can't* have a baby. My daughter is evidence to the contrary!)

But—there's always a but—I gained 50 pounds in the process. It was a huge struggle to lose the extra weight. My hormones went wild after the delivery, setting off a case of postpartum blues, hair loss, and extreme fatigue. I also waged a six-month touch-and-go struggle to breastfeed, which I detail here in the book.

I had a second pregnancy at 40, which ended in a miscarriage at 10 weeks. My progesterone levels were simply not high enough to support the pregnancy, apparently. Losing a baby at any point in a pregnancy is such a heartbreak.

Now, at 44, I'm mother to a second child: we adopted a precious little boy in 2005. It's wonderful, but very tiring, to have a little one again! But one other thing is making me tired—I'm in perimenopause. Truly, it's a challenge to stay balanced given the ups and downs of my hormones.

So, all along the way, from my efforts to get pregnant more than nine years ago to my current adventures with perimenopause, I've had to immerse myself in information on women's hormones, fertility, pregnancy, postpartum health, and the endocrine system in order to understand and meet my own challenges. The result is this book, written for the millions of you who, like me, are riding the hormonal roller coaster!

Many of you don't even know you have a thyroid problem. I hope this book can provide a road map that will help you move quickly through the process of recognizing your symptoms, getting diagnosed, and receiving proper treatment.

Many of you have already been diagnosed and treated for a thyroid condition. But if your thyroid treatment is not optimized and carefully monitored, you are opening yourself up to a number of hormonal complaints. For example, during the time you are trying to become pregnant, and during early pregnancy, proper thyroid treatment and oversight can make the difference between infertility or miscarriage and a successful pregnancy and healthy baby.

For example, Mandy has been hypothyroid since she had radioactive iodine treatment, and now she has many unresolved hormonal symptoms.

> I have gained weight. Diet and exercise have produced little positive result. I have uterine fibroids that cause extremely heavy periods. So much so that for at least two days of the month, I am very limited in the activities that I can participate in, as I bleed through double/super protection in 30 minutes. This was not so before thyroid disease. I have a much lower sex drive. My interest level is dramatically different now than during hyperthyroid days. My partner of 10 years is exasperated and is talking about leaving. I became pregnant and miscarried at one point. I do not even entertain the idea that pregnancy is an option for me anymore.

There is no reason that women like Mandy should have to suffer with symptoms like this. I also hope that some of you reading this book are practitioners trying to better understand your patients. More than ever, your patients are struggling with the implications of hormonal imbalances. There's a dizzying array of options—with everything from a birth control pill that lets you have only 4 menstrual periods a year, fertility treatments that allow women to get pregnant well into their forties and fifties, and pills, powders, and potions that all promise to solve the symptoms of menopause now that the old standby, Premarin, has fallen out of favor.

I can't promise that thyroid treatment is the solution for every woman struggling with PMS, fertility, menopause, or other hormonal challenges. But it is a solution for some, and the benefits of diagnosis and proper treatment are immeasurable.

# Part I

# THE THYROID

# Chapter 1

# About the Thyroid and Thyroid Disease

The reasonable man adapts himself to the world;
the unreasonable one persists in trying to
adapt the world to himself.
Therefore all progress depends on the unreasonable man.
—George Bernard Shaw

The normal thyroid is a small gland weighing about an ounce that sits behind the Adam's apple in the lower part of the neck, in front of the windpipe.

It derives its name from the Greek word *thyreoeides*, meaning "shield-shaped." In fact, it looks like a bowtie or butterfly, with the two "wings," or lobes, of the gland connected in the middle by the isthmus.

The thyroid, like other glands, is a discrete soft body made up of a large number of vessels that produce, store, and release—or secrete—some substance. Some glands secrete their products outside the body, some inside. Those that secrete hormones and metabolic substances on the inside of the body are known as *endocrine glands*. The endocrine glands include the thyroid, the parathyroids, the adrenal gland, the pancreas, the pituitary gland, the pineal gland, the gonads (ovaries and testes), and the thymus.

Doctors who specialize in treating patients with endocrine problems—disorders of the endocrine glands—are called *endocrinologists.*

*Hormones* are internal secretions carried in the blood to various organs. The thyroid's main purpose is to produce, store, and release two key hormones: triiodothyronine, also called T3; and thyroxine, or T4. The numbers 3 and 4 refer to the number of iodine molecules attached to each hormone.

Thyroid cells are the primary cells in the body capable of absorbing iodine, an essential nutrient. The thyroid takes in iodine, obtained through food, iodized salt, or supplements, and combines that iodine with the amino acid tyrosine, converting them to T3 and T4.

A healthy thyroid produces about 20 percent T3 and 80 percent T4. T3 is the biologically active hormone that is used by the cells; it is several times stronger than T4. As needed, the body converts the inactive T4 to active T3 by removing one iodine molecule. This conversion process is called *monodeiodination.* This conversion can take place in certain organs other than the thyroid, including the hypothalamus, a part of your brain.

T3 and T4 both exist in two forms: unbound and bound. Unbound, or free, T3 or T4 are biologically active; bound T3 and T4 are attached to the thyroid-binding globulin (TBG) protein. When measured in the blood, the free, or unbound, T3 and T4 levels tend to be most representative of the actual hormone available for use by the body.

The role of your thyroid hormones is to control your metabolism—the process by which oxygen and calories are converted to energy for use by your cells and organs. There's not a single cell in your body that doesn't depend on thyroid hormone for regulation and for energy in some form. And the thyroid hormones have a number of functions as they travel through the bloodstream. They

Enable cells to convert oxygen and calories into energy
Help the body process carbohydrates
Aid in the proper functioning of muscles
Enable proper sexual development and functioning
Help the heart pump properly and effectively
Help the body to breathe normally
Help the intestinal system digest and eliminate food
Strengthen hair, nails, and skin
Help the brain to function properly
Help with normal bone growth

Now that you have some idea of what the thyroid is and its location and function, let's go into more detail about how it fits into the overall functioning of the body.

## The Thyroid Gland: Setting the Pace

When your thyroid works normally, it produces and secretes the amount of T3 and T4 necessary to keep various body functions moving at their proper pace. However, the thyroid does not do this alone. It works as part of a bigger system, one that includes the pituitary gland and the hypothalamus.

Here's how the system works. The hypothalamus constantly monitors the pace of many of the body's functions. It also monitors and reacts to a number of other factors, including environmental factors such as heat, cold, and stress. If the hypothalamus senses that certain adjustments are needed to react to any of these factors, then it produces thyrotropin-releasing hormone, known as TRH.

TRH is sent from the hypothalamus to the pituitary gland. The pituitary gland is stimulated to produce a substance called thyrotropin, but better known as thyroid-stimulating hormone, or TSH for short. The pituitary gland also monitors the body and can release TSH based on the thyroid hormone levels circulating in your blood.

TSH is sent to the thyroid gland, where it causes the thyroid to produce, store, and release more T3 and T4 thyroid hormones.

The released thyroid hormones move into the bloodstream, carried by a plasma protein known as thyroxine-binding globulin (TBG).

Now in the bloodstream, the thyroid hormone travels throughout the body, carrying orders to the various organs. Upon arriving at a particular tissue in the body, thyroid hormones interact with receptors located inside the nucleus of the cells. Interaction of the hormone and the receptor will trigger a certain function, giving directions to that tissue regarding the rate at which it should operate.

When the hypothalamus senses that the need for increased thyroid hormone production has ended, it reduces production of TRH. The reduced production of TRH in turn causes the pituitary to decrease production of TSH, and the reduced TSH levels send the message to the gland itself to slow production of thyroid hormone. By this system, many of the body's organs keep working at the proper pace.

Think of the entire feedback loop as somewhat like the thermostat in your house. It's set to maintain a particular temperature, and when it detects that your house has become too hot, it signals to either stop blowing heat (or start blowing air conditioning). And when the house becomes too cold, the heat will kick on (or the air conditioning will turn off). In similar fashion, your body is set to maintain a certain level of circulating thyroid hormone.

When thyroid disease or other conditions interfere with the system and the feedback process doesn't work, however, thyroid problems can develop.

## Prevalence of Thyroid Disorders

Thyroid problems are widespread around the world. It is estimated that more than 200 million people worldwide have thyroid disease. Thyroid problems are particularly common in areas covered at one time by glaciers, where iodine is not present in the soil and in foods. In many of these countries, as many as one in five people have an enlarged thyroid, known as goiter, usually due to iodine deficiency. According to the World Health Organization, iodine deficiency is the world's most prevalent—yet easily preventable—cause of brain damage. It affects more than 780 million people worldwide—13 percent of the world's population. As many as an additional 30 percent of the population worldwide is at risk of iodine deficiency-related problems.

Pregnant women with mild iodine deficiency may give birth to children with moderate cognitive and developmental problems—a reduction in IQ of as much as 15 points. Serious iodine deficiency during pregnancy can cause stillbirth, miscarriage, on a congenital abnormality known as cretinism. Cretinism is a severe, irreversible form of mental retardation, and is most common in iodine-deficient areas of Africa and Asia.

In the United States and countries where iodine deficiency is not rampant, other types of thyroid problems are more common, especially the autoimmune disorder known as Hashimoto's disease. According to the latest diagnostic standards, there are some 54 million people in the United States with thyroid conditions. In the United States, only one in five people with thyroid conditions are actually being treated, however.

In the United States, the majority of thyroid conditions are due to autoimmune disease. The prevalence of thyroid disease increases with age. American women face a one-in-five chance of developing a thyroid problem. Women are seven to eight times more likely than men to develop thyroid conditions.

Besides iodine deficiency and being a woman, other risk factors include genetics and heredity, personal or family history of endocrine or autoimmune disease, infection, exposure to goitrogenic foods, cigarette smoking, pregnancy, certain drugs, particular chemical exposures, and radiation exposure. The risk factors are outlined in detail in Chapter 5.

## Thyroid Conditions

There are a number of conditions that can affect the thyroid's function and structure.

### Hypothyroidism or Underactive Thyroid

Hypothyroidism means there is too little thyroid hormone. It can result from a thyroid that is not producing enough hormone, has been radioactively ablated, is affected by drugs or nutritional deficiencies, or is incapable of functioning properly due to nodules, infection, or atrophy. When all or part of the thyroid is removed—as a treatment for cancer, nodules, goiter, Graves' disease, or hyperthyroidism—the vast majority of patients become permanently hypothyroid. A small number of infants are born without a thyroid, or without a functioning thyroid; this is known as congenital hypothyroidism.

Symptoms of hypothyroidism include fatigue, weight gain, constipation, fuzzy thinking, depression, body pain, slow reflexes, and much more.

Conventional treatment typically involves replacing the missing thyroid hormone using prescription thyroid hormone replacement drugs. Most commonly, a levothyroxine (T4) drug is prescribed, as this is considered the "standard" treatment for hypothyroidism. The most popular levothyroxine drug with physicians is Synthroid, and the term Synthroid is sometimes used to describe "thyroid hormone replacement drugs" (in the same way that the brand name Kleenex has become synonymous with "tissue"). This popularity is mainly due to extensive marketing by the manufacturer, however, and all the brand name levothyroxine drugs (Synthroid, Levoxyl, Levothroid, Unithroid, etc.) are considered to be similar in quality, potency, and effectiveness. Note, however, that Levoxyl has a fast-dissolving formula; it should be taken with plenty of water and swallowed quickly so as to maximize absorption.

Research has shown that many patients feel better with the addition of T3, so increasing numbers of practitioners are prescribing either Cytomel—liothyronine—or, less commonly, levothyroxine plus compounded T3.

Another option is a synthetic T4-T3 combination drug known as liotrix (brand name Thyrolar). While this drug is not commonly prescribed, it is a safe and effective option for some patients.

From the early 1900s to the 1950s, the only form of thyroid replacement drug available was natural thyroid, which was marketed under the brand name Armour Thyroid. The drug fell out of favor with some endocrinologists in the second half of the twentieth century as a result of Synthroid's extensive marketing efforts. However, since the 1990s, Armour Thyroid has been enjoying a resurgence in popularity with some patients and practitioners. Derived from the desiccated thyroid gland of pigs, the drug contains natural forms of numerous thyroid hormones and nutrients typically found in the actual thyroid gland, and some patients report greater improvement in symptoms using natural thyroid.

Where the thyroid is not surgically removed or chemically deactivated, holistic and integrative treatments focus on support for better thyroid and immune system function, enhancing metabolism and rebalancing the endocrine and hormonal systems through nutrition, herbs, supplements, movement therapy such as yoga, and energy work.

## Hyperthyroidism or Overactive Thyroid

Hyperthyroidism—too much throid hormone—can result in thyrotoxicosis. Hyperthyroidism can be caused by a number of thyroid problems, including autoimmune Graves' disease, nodules that produce thyroid hormone, overdosage of thyroid hormone replacement drugs, or infection. It is typically treated by drugs that reduce the thyroid's ability to produce hormone, by radioactive iodine treatment to chemically ablate the thyroid, or by surgery.

Symptoms of hyperthyroidism tend to mirror the rapid metabolism that results from an oversupply of thyroid hormone: anxiety, insomnia, rapid weight loss, diarrhea, high heart rate, high blood pressure, eye sensitivity or bulging, vision disturbances, and many other concerns.

Here how Janine describes her hyperthyroidism symptoms:

I started to feel weird, spacey, not feeling right in the head, anxious, heart palpitations, shaky, irritable, lost my appetite, trembling body, losing weight, sweating in the night and not sleeping, and wondering what in God's name was wrong with me. I had dizziness and shakiness, my heart pounding, tingling in my right arm and on my right cheek. I knew there was something wrong.

The anxiety of hyperthyroidism can sometimes be so significant that it is mistaken for anxiety or panic disorder. Kelly describes the anxiety of thyroid disease:

I felt like I was on an airplane that was about to crash with uncontrollable, impending doom.

Conventional treatment in the United States focuses on disabling the thyroid permanently by administering radioactive iodine (RAI) treatment, which renders most patients hypothyroid for life. Some physicians use prescription antithyroid drugs such as propylthiouracil (PTU) and methimazole (Tapazole) and beta blockers to calm down the thyroid and the immune system, with the hope of remission of the disease, which occurs in as many as 30 percent of patients. Antithyroid drugs are the first choice for doctors outside the United States. In rare cases in the United States, and more commonly outside the United States, surgery to remove the thyroid may be the treatment. Holistic and integrative treatments prior to RAI or surgery focus on supplementing antithyroid drug approaches with natural antithyroid foods, supplements, and herbs that have no side effects, as well as calming and rebalancing the immune system through nutrition, herbs, supplements, movement therapy such as yoga, and energy work.

Ultimately, most people with hyperthyroidism do end up hypothyroid for life as a result of RAI or surgery.

### Goiter

Goiter is the term used to describe an enlargement of the thyroid gland. The thyroid gland can enlarge as a response to deficiencies of iodine, thyroid inflammation or infection, or autoimmune disease. The thyroid becomes large enough that it can be seen as enlarged by ultrasound or X-ray, and may be enlarged enough to thicken the neck area visibly. Particularly large goiters may be cosmetically problematic, and can compromise breathing and swallowing; they are often surgically removed. Smaller goiters may respond to drug treatment.

Symptoms of goiter include a swollen, tender, or tight feeling in the neck or throat; hoarseness or coughing; and difficulty swallowing or breathing.

Goiter can be due to an autoimmune condition that triggers an inflamed thyroid, or too much or too little iodine in the diet. In the United States, 10 to 20 percent of goiters are iodine-induced.

Treatment for goiter depends on how enlarged the thyroid has become, as well as other symptoms. Treatments can include:

- Observation and monitoring, which is typically done if the goiter is not large and is not causing symptoms or thyroid dysfunction.
- Medications, including thyroid hormone replacement, which can help shrink the goiter, or aspirin or corticosteroid drugs, to shrink thyroid inflammation.
- If the goiter is very large, continues to grow despite drug therapy, is in a dangerous location (blocking the

windpipe or esophagus), or becomes cosmetically un-sightly, most doctors will recommend surgery. If the goi-ter contains any suspicious nodules, surgery may also be necessary.

### Nodules or Lumps

Many people have nodules in the thyroid, but few are pal-pable (capable of being felt externally). Thyroid nodules are actually fairly common. An estimated 1 in 12 to 15 women and 1 in 50 men has a thyroid nodule. In some cases, nodules on the thyroid exist without any disease, don't have any active function, and cause no symptoms. Some nodules impair the thyroid's ability to function properly and cause hypothyroid-ism. In some cases, nodules are overactive and produce far too much thyroid hormone; these are called "toxic nodules," and can trigger hyperthyroidism. Particularly large nodules can compromise breathing or swallowing. A very small percent-age of nodules are cancerous. In nonpregnant patients, 90 to 95 percent of nodules are benign. In pregnant women, how-ever, approximately 27 percent of nodules are cancerous.

Some people will have no symptoms, while others may have hyperthyroid symptoms such as palpitations, insomnia, weight loss, anxiety, and tremors. Nodules can also trigger hypothy-roidism, and symptoms might include weight gain, fatigue, or depression. Some people will cycle back and forth between hyperthyroid and hypothyroid symptoms. Others may have difficulty swallowing; a feeling of fullness, pain, or pressure in the neck; a hoarse voice; or neck tenderness. And finally, many people have nodules with no obvious symptoms related to thy-roid dysfunction at all.

Depending on the results of the evaluation, nodules may be left alone and monitored periodically, assuming they aren't

causing serious difficulty, or treated with thyroid hormone replacement to help shrink them. They will be surgically removed
if they are causing difficulties with breathing or if test results
indicate a suspected malignancy.

## Thyroid Diseases

A variety of diseases affect the thyroid and trigger thyroid conditions such as hypothyroidism, hyperthyroidism, nodules, or
goiter.

### Autoimmune Thyroid Disease

There are two different autoimmune diseases in which an immune system dysfunction targets the thyroid: Graves' disease
and Hashimoto's disease. In the United States, the vast majority of thyroid patients are either hypothyroid or hyperthyroid
due to an autoimmune disease.

Hashimoto's disease is the most common form of thyroiditis, an inflammation of the thyroid, so the condition is often
referred to as Hashimoto's thyroiditis. It is far more common
than Graves' disease, and is the cause of most hypothyroidism
in the United States. In Hashimoto's, antibodies react against
proteins in the thyroid, causing gradual destruction of the
gland itself. Occasionally, before the thyroid is destroyed, it has
thyrotoxic periods—known as hashitoxicosis—during which
the thyroid overproduces thyroid hormone. Eventually, however, the gland's attack on itself destroys the ability to produce
the thyroid hormones the body needs.

Symptoms of Hashimoto's disease usually parallel the
hypothyroidism that results; however, the thyroid can periodically sputter into life during hashitoxic periods, causing symp-

toms of hyperthyroidism. For most people, treatment is for hypothyroidism and involves lifelong thyroid hormone replacement. Holistic and integrative approaches tend to look at healing the underlying autoimmune imbalance, and may include nutritional support for the thyroid (i.e., selenium, tyrosine, B vitamins, etc.) and overall support for the immune system.

Graves' disease—sometimes referred to as "diffuse toxic goiter" because of the usual presence of a goiter—typically causes hyperthyroidism. Graves' disease and hyperthyroidism appear to affect slightly less than 1 percent of the U.S. population, or slightly fewer than 2.9 million people. Some experts believe, however, that as many as 4 percent of Americans, or 11.8 million people, may have a mild, subclinical form of Graves' disease; they have few or no symptoms but exhibit blood-test evidence of slight hyperthyroidism.

In Graves' disease, antibodies bind to the gland, which causes the thyroid to overproduce hormone, resulting in hyperthyroidism. Treatment for Graves' disease follows hyperthyroidism treatment: antithyroid drugs, radioactive iodine ablation, or surgical removal of the thyroid. Most Graves' disease patients end up hypothyroid over time, requiring lifelong thyroid hormone replacement.

### Thyroid Cancer

Thyroid cancer is one of the least common cancers in the United States, but it is the most common form of endocrine cancer. The incidence of thyroid cancer is on the rise in recent years in the United States. The American Cancer Society estimated that there were almost 26,000 new cases of thyroid cancer in 2005 (some 19,200 occurring in women); an estimated 1,500 people died of thyroid cancer in 2005.

Treatment and prognosis depend on the type of thyroid cancer. Papillary and follicular thyroid cancer are the most common types; an estimated 80 to 90 percent of all thyroid cancers fall into this category. Most papillary and follicular thyroid cancer can be treated successfully when discovered early. Medullary thyroid carcinoma (MTC) makes up 5 to 10 percent of all thyroid cancers. If discovered before it metastasizes to other parts of the body, medullary cancer has a good cure rate. There are two types of medullary thyroid cancer: sporadic and familial. Anyone with a family history of MTC should take a blood test to measure high calcitonin levels, which may indicate a strong genetic predisposition. If high level are found, many people decide to undergo a thyroidectomy—surgical removal of the thyroid—as a preventive measure. Anaplastic thyroid carcinoma is quite rare, accounting for only 1 to 2 percent of all thyroid cancers. It tends to be quite aggressive and is the least likely to respond to typical methods of treatment.

Although many patients are asymptomatic at first, possible symptoms of thyroid cancer include a lump in the neck, voice changes, difficulty breathing or swallowing, or lymph node swelling.

Treatment for thyroid cancer almost always involves surgery to remove the thyroid and the cancer. In some cases, cancerous lymph nodes in the neck may be removed. Radiation therapy is typically used to kill any remaining cancer cells. Radiation for thyroid cancer is commonly administered by ingestion of liquid radioactive iodine (RAI). Because the thyroid takes up iodine, the radioactive iodine collects in any thyroid tissue remaining in the body and kills the cancer cells. Less commonly, external radiation therapy may be given. Hormone therapy, using thyroid hormone, is often used to stop cancer cells from growing.

Because the entire thyroid is removed as treatment for most thyroid cancers, almost all thyroid cancer survivors end up hypothyroid, and need to take thyroid replacement hormone for life. Their medication needs to be at a high enough dose to ensure that their TSH levels remain low—nearly undetectable, actually—to help prevent a relapse of cancer. Survivors need regular checks to watch for a recurrence.

## Thyroiditis

While Hashimoto's disease is by far the most common form of thyroiditis, there are other forms. These include:

- De Quervain's thyroiditis, granulomatous thyroiditis, painful thyroiditis, or subacute thyroiditis: a viral thyroiditis that can have a thyrotoxic phase
- Painless thyroiditis (also known as silent thyroiditis and lymphocytic thyroiditis): a temporary thyroid condition that may involve mild hyperthyroidism during its thyrotoxic phase, followed by a period of hypothyroidism and a return to normal
- Postpartum thyroiditis: a form of painless or silent thyroiditis that affects 5 to 10 percent of women within a year of giving birth; it typically starts out with a thyrotoxic period of hyperthyroidism
- Acute suppurative thyroiditis: a rare situation where the thyroid is infected with bacteria and abscessed

Thyroiditis typically includes pain and tenderness in the thyroid area, neck, and throat, as well as difficulty sleeping. It may also manifest with either hypothyroid or hyperthyroid symptoms.

Treatment depends on the manifestation of thyroiditis, and may include a short course of antithyroid drugs or beta blockers if hyperthyroid, thyroid hormone replacement for hypothyroidism, or antibiotics for a suppurative thyroiditis. If the main symptom is pain, nonsteroidal anti-inflammatory drugs like ibuprofen (Motrin, Advil) or naproxen (Aleve) may be helpful.

### Ending Up Hypothyroid

Whatever the thyroid disease or condition, most thyroid patients end up hypothyroid in the end, because the treatments for thyroid conditions such as hyperthyroidism, Graves' disease, nodules, goiter, and thyroid cancer almost always curtail or eliminate thyroid function, leaving patients unable to produce sufficient thyroid hormone on their own. In addition, most people with Hashimoto's disease, the most common thyroid condition, eventually become hypothyroid as the gland is gradually destroyed by the autoimmune process.

The holistic medical community feels that hypothyroidism is underestimated, and that we are actually undergoing an epidemic. Some physicians believe that as many as 40 to 60 percent of the population are suffering from some form of hypothyroidism.

# Chapter 2

## Women's Hormones

> If women are supposed to be less rational and more emotional at
> the beginning of our menstrual cycle when the female hormone
> is at its lowest level, then why isn't it logical to say that, in those
> few days, women behave the most like the way men behave all
> month long?
>
> —Gloria Steinem

In order to understand how your thyroid and hormones all
work together, you first need to understand the endocrine
system.

The endocrine system handles reproduction, growth, metabolism, energy, nutritional balance, stressors, and a number
of other essential functions. There are eight different endocrine
glands in the system.

- Ovaries in women; testes in men
- Adrenal gland
- Pancreatic islets
- Thyroid gland
- Parathyroid gland

- Pineal gland
- Pituitary gland
- Hypothalamus

The endocrine system also includes cells in the stomach, heart, and a number of other organs that produce hormones.

The hypothalamus, which is located in the brain, is also part of the nervous system and provides a critical link between the endocrine and nervous systems. It acts as the endocrine system's primary coordinator and command center, releasing hormones to help control the other glands' activities and acting to coordinate the various glands and hormonal cycles.

A key hypothalamic function is its effect on the body's stress response. The hypothalamus causes the pituitary to release hormones that cause the adrenals to release stress hormones.

The hypothalamus also releases the hormone that causes the pituitary to stimulate the ovaries to develop egg follicles and set the female menstual cycle in motion.

## Reproductive Hormonal Cycle

To understand the relationship between the thyroid and various hormonal conditions that affect women, it's also essential to understand exactly how the reproductive hormonal cycle works. Many of us think we understand: The egg develops, uterine lining builds up, egg is released, if the egg isn't fertilized, the lining is shed, and that's your period. Then the whole thing starts again. But a much more sophisticated hormonal interaction keeps the whole cycle moving and in balance.

The female reproductive cycle involves a continuous feedback loop between the brain and the ovaries, and the hormones that each produce. The command center for the body's reproductive and endocrine systems is the hypothalamus, located in the brain. Some people describe it as a kind of thermostat, turning up and down the levels of various hormones and chemicals in the body.

The hypothalamus produces a number of hormones, but the key one for reproduction is gonadotropin-releasing hormone (GnRH). Typically, GnRH is released in "pulses" every one to two hours.

GnRH communicates with the body's master gland, the pituitary, also located in the brain. The pituitary gland's function is to send out various hormones and transmitters to control the activities of other glands.

For reproduction, the pituitary, stimulated by GnRH, produces two key hormones: follicle-stimulating hormone (FSH), which triggers follicles (eggs) to develop in the ovaries and causes estrogen to rise; and luteinizing hormone (LH), which helps with the development and maturation of eggs and causes ovulation.

FSH and LH also communicate with the ovaries and the corpus luteum. The ovaries produce estrogen, and the corpus luteum produces progesterone. Changes in estrogen and progesterone are involved in preparing the uterine lining for possible pregnancy and in triggering the onset of menstruation, among many other important functions.

The process is depicted in the Figure 1. The relationship of key hormones is sometimes referred to as the hormonal cascade, meaning that each hormone is a controller or precursor for the next hormone downstream. This is particularly evident in looking at reproductive hormones, most of which fall into the steroid category.

The building block of reproductive hormones is actually cholesterol, which becomes the primary reproductive hormone, pregnenolone, which is produced in the adrenal glands. Preg-

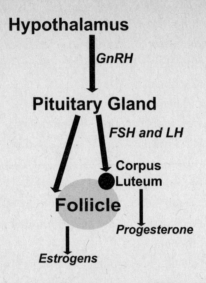

*FIGURE 1: THE HORMONAL CASCADE*

nenolone is the precursor for all the key steroid hormones. Directed by the brain, it is converted in the ovaries, testes, and adrenal glands into these key steroid hormones:

- DHEA, which is metabolized into DHEA-sulfate (DHEA-S), the type of DHEA usually measured because it is fairly stable.
- Testosterone
- The estrogens: estrone (E1), estradiol (E2), and estriol (E3)
- Progesterone
- Cortisol

The steroid hormones, estrogen and progesterone in particular, travel to various tissues, organs, and glands, some of which have receptors for these particular hormones. The hormone enters the cell, binds to and activates the receptor, which then sets various physiological processes into motion.

Dr. Sherrill Sellman explains their importance:

> What is often misunderstood when we talk about the hor-mones estrogen and progesterone is the fact that they aren't just about overseeing reproduction. There are, in fact, recep-tor sites for both these hormones in every cell throughout the body. Thus the immune system, the nervous system, the circulatory system, the digestive system, the vascular system, the respiratory system all are affected by the flow and proper balance between these two hormones.

## Puberty

When a girl is born, her ovaries contain hundreds of thousands of immature eggs. These are all the eggs she will ever have. Over time, eggs mature and are released, while others die with-out maturing.

Around age 8 to 10 the female body starts producing andro-gens, which trigger the onset of puberty. The start of puberty is usually signaled by breast development and the appearance of pubic and underarm hair.

Vaginal discharge can also appear, typically around six months before the first period.

The first menstrual period often occurs approximately two to two and a half years after puberty starts, but it can start as early as a year, and as late as three years. Typically, the first menstrual period will take place when a girl is around 100 pounds and has approximately 25 percent body fat; some ex-perts consider these to be the body's minimum weight and level of fat reserves to support and sustain a pregnancy. This hap-pens, on average, around age 12 to 13 for most girls.

The process that triggers the first menstrual period begins when the hypothalamus sends out the first burst of gonadotrophin-releasing hormone (GnRH). GnRH goes to the pituitary gland, where it triggers the pituitary to release two hormones: luteinizing hormone (LH) and follicle-stimulating hormone (FSH). FSH and LH stimulate the ovaries to begin producing estrogen. Estrogen, FSH, and LH then set into motion the hormonal cycle that causes the ovary to ovulate—to release its first egg. This begins the first menstrual cycle.

Through puberty, breasts typically develop further and the hair becomes thicker and heavier. This is also a time when body odor starts to appear. Hips typically widen somewhat, and the girl will usually go through a period of growth, with some weight gain as well.

## The Menstrual Cycle

After the onset of menstruation, a woman is in her menstruating years, which typically last 30 to 40 years. This is a time frame when some women have a fairly stable and consistent menstrual cycle. The period from the late teens to the late twenties is usually when a woman is at her most fertile. Fertility starts to declines in the thirties, declines even further as a woman reaches her forties, and the chance of becoming pregnant becomes much less as a woman moves into perimenopause.

Day 1 of the menstrual cycle starts the follicular phase of the menstrual cycle. During this phase, estrogen and progesterone are at their lowest levels. These low levels are a signal to the pituitary to begin the menstrual cycle by releasing FSH. As FSH rises, eggs mature, and fluid is collected around the eggs, creating follicles. The number of follicles that develop each month is unique to each woman.

Around day 10 of the cycle, one follicle becomes dominant and grows faster than the others. (Occasionally, with higher FSH levels, additional follicles may become dominant. This can cause multiple births.)

As the follicles grow, they release increasing amounts of estrogen. This estrogen causes the lining of the uterus to thicken over the next seven days. When FSH gets to its highest point and the estrogen produced by the follicles reaches a particular level, the estrogen levels trigger a rapid release—known as a surge—of luteinizing hormone (LH). This typically occurs around day 13 of the cycle. The level of LH is only high during the time an egg is being released. (The LH surge is what is measured by home ovulation detection kits.)

In the meantime, as estrogen levels have been increasing, the FSH decreases, and the nondominant follicles wither away and are reabsorbed.

As ovulation approaches, the fallopian tubes ready themselves for a fertilized egg. The rise in estrogen changes the cervical fluid, making it stringy, sticky, more friendly for sperm, and more conducive to conception. The cervix itself becomes softer and more open, also making conception more possible.

The LH surge, usually occurring on days 12 to 14, sets in motion the final maturation of the egg and causes the dominant follicle to force its way to the surface of the ovary, rupture, and release the egg into the fallopian tube—a process known as ovulation. Typically, ovulation occurs between 28 and 36 hours after the LH surge, and about 12 hours after LH reaches peak levels.

The days before ovulation are considered the most fertile days in the cycle for intercourse or insemination. Sperm typically survive as long as three days, and some survive for as many as seven days in a woman's body, so if sperm are introduced in the days before ovulation, it is likely that they will still be alive when the egg is released. The egg can live for about 20 hours after ovulation, so the day or two after ovulation are also considered fertile days.

As the egg is released, some women can feel a slight twinge in the lower back or abdomen. This is sometimes referred to as mittelschmerz, or middle pain. Some women have very slight spotting or discharge at ovulation as well.

After the egg is released, it is swept into the fallopian tube, where fertilization usually takes place.

The remaining components of the dominant follicle that were not ovulated are transformed into the corpus luteum, which produces high levels of progesterone and some estrogen; these are used to prepare the uterine lining for implantation of a fertilized egg (an embryo). This built-up uterine lining is known as the endometrium.

Ovulation signals the end of the follicular phase and the start of the luteal phase of the menstrual cycle. During this second half of the menstrual cycle, which normally runs anywhere from 12 to 15 days, the body attempts to support a pregnancy if one occurs.

If pregnancy does not occur, around 10 days after ovulation the corpus luteum starts to break down and slowly stops producing both progesterone and estrogen.

As estrogen and progesterone fall sharply, on days 26 to 28, the premenstrual phase begins. Premenstrual syndrome (PMS) is most common at this time.

When the follicle has self-destructed completely, the drop in progesterone triggers the shedding of the endometrium as menstrual bleeding, typically starting on day 28—about 14 days after ovulation.

The menstrual phase can last from one to eight days, but the average is four to five days. The length of the bleeding period tends to remain about the same in women from month to month, but over time it may become longer or shorter. The amount of blood lost in each menstruation tends to be similar from cycle to cycle in many women, but over time it can become heavier or lighter.

This first day of menstrual bleeding—often day 28 of the cycle—also triggers the pituitary to release FSH and start the cycle again. So day 28 is also day 1 of the new cycle.

When the entire system is working properly, the follicular phase—maturation of the egg—takes 14 days on average, and the corpus luteum—which defines the luteal phase—has a life span of approximately 14 days. Thus, a typical menstrual cycle is 28 days, with ovulation occurring around the midpoint on day 14.

- Day 1: Menstrual period begins.
- Days 1–14: Follicular phase.
- Day 14: Ovulation.
- Days 14–28: Luteal phase.
- Days 26–28: Premenstrual phase.
- Day 28 (day 1): Menstrual period begins.

Each woman's cycle is unique and may not fit this "typical" 28-day cycle. The normal cycle can range from as little as 21 days to 40 or more days. For most women, however, the luteal phase lasts about 12 to 16 days. If a woman has a particularly long cycle, the additional time will usually extend the length of the follicular phase.

## Pregnancy

During pregnancy, there is a virtual symphony of hormones, working in concert to assure the viability of the pregnancy.

## Human Chorionic Gonadotropin

When the egg is fertilized, it sends out a hormone called human chorionic gonadotropin, or HCG. The HCG causes the corpus luteum to continue to make progesterone until around 10 weeks gestation, when the placenta takes over. Home pregnancy tests measure the level of HCG in the urine, and beta HCG blood tests measure HCG in the blood.

HCG is thought to play a part in causing characteristic symptoms of early pregnancy, including nausea, vomiting, and fatigue. HCG's main function is to communicate to the ovaries to produce progesterone to support the pregnancy until the placenta is formed, around week 10, when the placenta can take over progesterone production. HCG also prevents release of eggs from the ovaries.

There is evidence that HCG may interact with and stimulate the thyroid, both of the mother and of the fetus. The evidence is largely circumstantial, but researchers point to studies of thyroid tests in normal pregnancy, and the inverse relationship between HCG and TSH levels. Some believe that both HCG and TSH may be controlling the thyroid in early pregnancy.

## Progesterone

Both the ovaries and the placenta produce progesterone in pregnancy. Progesterone helps the uterine lining thicken in preparation for implantation after conception. Progesterone levels rise during pregnancy, and the progesterone aids in placental development and maintenance.

Progesterone inhibits contractions of the smooth muscles of the uterus, which protects the growing fetus. Progesterone also causes cartilage in the pelvis, hips, and public area to soften (to allow for widening of the birth canal during birth). Progesterone can also cause breast tenderness and a bloated feeling throughout pregnancy.

At the end of the pregnancy, the levels of progesterone drop, and it is this decrease that signals the start of labor, helping to stimulate contractions that will lead to birth.

## Estrogen

Estrogen, usually produced by the ovaries, is also produced by the placenta during pregnancy, with the levels increasing steadily until the baby is born. Estrogen helps increase blood flow to the uterus and regulate progesterone production. Estrogen also triggers proper organ development and prepares the breasts for lactation. Estrogen can cause tender and enlarged breasts, and fluctuating emotions, which are common symptoms of early pregnancy. Increasing estrogen levels also stimulate production of the hormone prolactin.

## Prostaglandins

Certain prostaglandins help soften the cervix and cause uterine contractions; levels of these hormones rise at the onset of labor. Oxytocin is released as a response when the cervix is stretched, as in delivery, and when the nipples are stimulated, as in breastfeeding. It helps make the uterus contract rapidly and stimulates the mammary glands to produce milk. (The contractions that some women feel while breastfeeding are due to oxytocin.) High levels of progesterone during pregnancy inhibit oxytocin from working, but when progesterone levels drop dramatically before birth, the oxytocin has its impact. Synthetic prostaglandins—Pitocin (synthetic oxytocin), and Cytotec (misoprostol)—are used to induce labor in a pregnancy that has gone past week 40.

## Prolactin

Prolactin is a hormone that typically increases during the late stage of pregnancy and remains elevated during the period of breastfeeding. Prolactin, produced by the pituitary gland, helps prepare the breasts for breastfeeding by increasing the milk-producing cells within the breasts. Progesterone and estrogen actually prevent milk production, so when these hormone levels drop immediately after birth, this stimulates the initial production of milk. Prolactin levels also inhibit pregnancy, but don't necessarily prevent it.

## Other Key Hormones

The following are some other pregnancy hormones:

- HPL (human placental lactogen) is produced in the placenta and helps the breasts develop milk-producing glands. The levels increase steadily through pregnancy until the last month of pregnancy.
- Calcitonin is a protein-based hormone that helps regulate bone development.
- Insulin helps the fetus store food and regulate both maternal and fetal glucose levels.
- Relaxin encourages the cervix and the pelvic muscles to relax, easing labor and birth.

# Postpartum Hormones

After delivery, progesterone and estrogen levels rapidly decrease, dropping by 90 percent within the first few days after birth. This sudden decline of hormones triggers the release of prolactin and oxytocin, to allow for breastfeeding.

After pregnancy, the stress hormone cortisol tends to rise. Research has actually shown that women with higher postpartum cortisol levels are more attentive to their babies, more attracted to their scent, and more responsive and inter-active—and therefore bonded—with their babies.

Oxytocin released during breastfeeding, however, appears to modulate the stress hormones—including cortisol, adreno-corticotropin, and vasopressin. This may make a woman who is lactating more resilient to stress.

## Perimenopause and Menopause

Perimenopause typically starts when a woman is in her late thirties, though it can begin earlier. As progesterone and estro-gen levels start to drop, this results in

- Increased FSH and LH levels
- More anovulatory cycles
- Skipped periods and periodic amenorrhea

As the key reproductive hormones decline, periods often become irregular. Low estrogen can make the vaginal walls thinner, which may make the vagina feel dry or irritated. The bladder lining also thins, which can contribute to more fre-quent urination, more urinary tract infections, or even inconti-nence. Fluctuating hormones can also worsen PMS symptoms and disturb sleep.

Eventually, as hormones continue to decline, there are more anovulatory cycles. Because follicles don't develop, progester-one doesn't rise. This usually results in a reduction in PMS symptoms. New symptoms can start, however, including hot flashes and night sweats. As hormone levels drop further, bleed-ing tends to become heavier and longer, and is brown rather than red. Periods can become more erratic, and with more anovulatory cycles, more missed periods can be expected.

Menopause, signaling the depletion of egg stocks, usually arrives between the ages of 45 and 55, and is defined as the point one year after the last menstrual period.

By the time menopause is official, production of estrogen and progesterone has fallen by 90 percent.

## Thyroid and Reproductive Hormones

The thyroid is a key player in the endocrine and reproductive hormonal cycles. It has an impact on these cycles in a number of important ways.

First, thyroid hormone regulates metabolism, and as such, it controls the functions and activities of your cells. At the most basic level, if the thyroid is not functioning properly, the cell's ability to use energy and perform essential functions in organs and glands throughout the body, including the reproductive system, is compromised.

Second, thyroid hormone is essential to the process of converting cholesterol into pregnenolone, and converting pregnenolone into progesterone, DHEA, estrogen, and testosterone. Any deficiency or excess of thyroid hormone can disrupt the entire hormone production process.

Third, thyroid hormone has some chemical similarities to estrogen and progesterone. The various receptor sites for thyroid, found throughout the body, can therefore be blocked—or helped—by the presence of estrogen and progesterone.

Dr. Glenn Rothfeld describes this process well in his useful book *Thyroid Balance:*

Estrogen, progesterone and thyroid hormone are configured so that excess amounts of one can block the receptiveness of the cells to the others. In underactive thyroid, estrogen molecules tend to take up residence in available thyroid receptors. They have no action when they do this, but they do keep thyroid hormone molecules from binding with the receptors. This prevents thyroid hormone from playing its role in metabolism, further slowing cell functions. Oral contraceptive estrogens and estrogen replacement therapy also have this effect. In overactive thyroid, the opposite occurs. Thyroid hormone molecules bind to estrogen receptors in the cells. This keeps estrogen from binding, and interferes with the hormonal cycle of fertility.

Fourth, as estrogen levels increase, the need for thyroid hormone may increase as well. For example, hypothyroid women who have increased estrogen levels, due to either pregnancy, estrogen replacement therapy, or phytoestrogen intake, may have worsening signs and symptoms of thyroid deficiency, yet their blood level tests may appear normal. These women may still need higher doses of thyroid replacement hormone in order to correct the underlying hypothyroidism, and offset estrogen's ability to bind thyroid hormone and prevent it from being usable to the body's cells.

Fifth, progesterone levels have an impact on thyroid function, but in an opposite way to estrogen. As progesterone levels go up, thyroid hormone requirements may drop. Sufficient progesterone is actually necessary to ensure adequate binding of T3, the active thyroid hormone. Progesterone also stimulates estrogen receptor sites, to ensure proper balance of estrogen levels. Progesterone can decrease levels of thyroxine-binding globulin (TBG), thereby increasing thyroid hormone levels in the blood.

## Hormonal Problems of Thyroid Patients

A number of hormonal problems that affect the menstrual cycle, reproduction, fertility, pregnancy, and menopause are more common in thyroid patients.

### Anovulation

One of the ways that thyroid conditions can interfere with other hormones and cause problems, including PMS and other menstrual problems, fertility issues, and menopausal symptoms, is by causing anovulatory cycles—cycles in which you don't ovulate. Even when you have an anovulatory cycle, you may still build up endometrial lining and have a menstrual period, but since no egg is released, hormones are erratic and pregnancy is not possible.

Even without a thyroid problem, many women have a few anovulatory cycles each year, but they are seen more often in younger women who have just started menstruating, women who are breastfeeding, women in their midthirties and older women in perimenopause, and women with thyroid disease, in particular, hypothyroidism.

According to Dr. John Lee, author of *What Your Doctor Doesn't Tell You About Menopause*, a number of things can cause anovulatory cycles.

- Adrenal exhaustion and stress
- Poor diet
- Environmental exposures
- Progesterone deficiency

Dr. Lee also believes that situations of chronic stress, where there are high levels of cortisol circulating on a long-term basis, can lead to overall hormone resistance in a number of areas, including thyroid, which may in part explain why thyroid patients have more anovulatory cycles than normal.

## Hyperprolactinemia

Hypothyroidism may also have an impact on ovulation, and therefore affect fertility, menstrual cycles, and menstrual symptoms. In hypothyroidism, thyrotropin-releasing hormone is released by the hypothalamus as a way to stimulate the pituitary gland to release TSH. The TSH then sends the message to the thyroid to produce more hormone. Unfortunately, elevated TRH can miscommunicate with the pituitary at times, and instead trigger the release of *other* pituitary hormones, including prolactin. Prolactin's role is to stimulate milk production by the breasts. Prolactin is secreted by the pituitary, and rises in women who are pregnant or breastfeeding. Excess prolactin is a condition known as hyperprolactinemia. (In rare cases, certain kidney problems or benign pituitary tumors may cause prolactin release, but it is most often caused by a thyroid imbalance.) Hyperprolactinemia can cause a variety of hormonal problems.

- Irregular ovulation
- Irregular menstruation and menstrual problems, including amenorrhea
- Galactorrhea: production of breast milk, or a milky discharge from the breast in a woman who is not breastfeeding

Treating the hypothyroidism with thyroid hormone can often correct prolactin levels and return them to normal.

For women who are trying to become pregnant and have elevated prolactin levels that are not caused by hypothyroidism, or are unresponsive to thyroid treatment, the drug bromocriptine (Parlodel) is typically prescribed. This drug suppresses prolactin production. Within six to eight weeks, a woman will typically begin to ovulate normally again and menstrual cycles will usually regulate.

## Luteal Phase Defect

When the thyroid is imbalanced, progesterone levels can also be affected. Insufficient progesterone can lead to a luteal phase defect. The luteal phase is the time after ovulation and before menstruation starts, during which the fertilized egg is nurtured and implanted in the uterus. A typical luteal phase lasts 12 to 16 days. Fertility requires a sufficient luteal phase, because if the luteal phase is too short, implantation cannot properly occur, and the fertilized egg instead ends up being removed from the body at the same time menstruation would occur. Because it comes at the time of the period, however, many women do not recognize it as a very early miscarriage, but mistakenly think it's a regular menstrual period.

Luteal phase defect due to low progesterone can affect both hypothyroid and hyperthyroid patients. In one study, progesterone levels of women with Graves' disease were measured before and after starting antithyroid drugs. These women, who had low progesterone levels prior to treatment, were again measured four months after starting the antithyroid drugs, and their progesterone levels were still low.

## Sex Hormone–Binding Globulin (SHBG) Imbalances

In women with hypothyroid conditions, sex hormone–binding globulin (SHBG) is often decreased. This can lead to excessively high estrogen levels, which can interfere with the proper follicle growth development, and with the FSH and LH surges needed for proper ovulation. Decreased SHBG can also lead to chronic estrogen excess or dominance, described in the next section. In hyperthyroidism, SHBG can be elevated, which then lowers progesterone, a situation that can also lead to estrogen dominance.

## Estrogen Dominance

Thyroid hormone and estrogen are hormones that actually have opposite actions. Estrogen can inhibit the thyroid's actions in the cells, and interferes with the thyroid's ability to bind to its receptors. Because estrogen can compete with thyroid hormone at the receptor sites, too much circulating estrogen, or a predominance of estrogen compared to progesterone, may block thyroid hormone from getting into the cells. Even with normal circulating levels of thyroid hormone, this can leave a woman functionally hypothyroid at the cellular level. This condition is known as estrogen dominance.

## Progesterone Deficiency

Low progesterone is considered more common in women with thyroid conditions. In part, progesterone deficiency can be a result of anovulatory cycles in women with thyroid problems. While thyroid problems can predispose a woman toward more anovulatory cycles, anovulatory cycles also increase with age and onset of perimenopause, leading to further progesterone deficiency.

Progesterone also acts to activate the body's estrogen receptor sites. This allows any excess estrogen to be "received" and locked up before it can interfere with other functions or lock into thyroid receptor sites and block thyroid hormone delivery. Low thyroid hormone often indicates low progesterone levels.

# Chapter 3

# Diagnosing Thyroid Conditions

I wish I could be half as sure of anything as some people are of everything.

—Gerald Barzan

Some physicians will tell you that diagnosing thyroid disease is easy: "Just one blood test and we'll find out what we need to know." While there are some instances where thyroid disease or a thyroid condition is fairly simple to identify, most cases are not quite that easy, particularly if you're dealing with a more subtle or borderline problem.

A thorough conventional medical evaluation for thyroid disease will include a complete review of your thyroid risk factors, family history, personal history, and symptoms. An examination and clinical evaluation should be conducted, followed by blood tests and any needed imaging tests. This combination of history, examination, clinical signs, blood work, and other medical tests should enable a good practitioner to make a sound diagnosis.

## Evaluation of Clinical Signs

In a clinical examination of your thyroid, your doctor should feel for thyroid enlargement, nodules, and masses in your neck area. He or she should also listen to your thyroid using a stethoscope. Your reflexes will be checked: hyperresponsive reflexes can be a sign of hyperthyroidism, and slow reflexes may point to hypothyroidism. Your skin, hair, and eyes will be examined for visible signs of a thyroid condition. Your heart rate, rhythm, and blood pressure will be checked. Your weight should be measured. The doctor should also, in physical examination, evaluate your lymph node areas (neck, underarm, groin) and your spleen.

These are the clinical signs your practitioner should look for in making a diagnosis of thyroid disease.

### Thyroid-Specific Signs

Your doctor will look for specific thyroid-related signs.

- Goiter: A common sign of thyroid problems is goiter, an enlargement of the thyroid. A goiter may be visible, palpable, or seen on imaging tests.
- Nodules: The doctor may be able to feel or even see nodules or lumps in your thyroid.
- "Thrill" on palpation: The doctor can feel increased blood flow in the thyroid.
- "Bruit" on palpation: With a stethoscope, the doctor can hear the sound of increased blood flow in the thyroid.

### Liver Irregularities

Your doctor will feel for an enlarged liver and look for evidence of jaundice in your skin tone.

## Heart and Circulation Irregularities

These are the irregularities your doctor will look for:

- Very high or very low blood pressure.
- Atypical sinus rhythm: a fast heart rate.
- Sinus tachycardia: a fast but regular heartbeat, over 100 bpm (normal heart rate is 70 to 80).
- Bradycardia: a very slow heart rate, under 60 bpm in a nonathlete.
- Ventricular tachycardia: rapid heartbeat, felt as palpitations and sometimes also pounding.
- Atrial fibrillation: The upper and lower chambers of the heart (atria and ventricles) aren't functioning properly; the atria are beating faster than the ventricles or there is an inconsistent rhythm.
- Mitral valve prolapse: felt as palpitations and heart flutters.

## Body Temperature

Your temperature should be measured, looking for two possible thyroid signs:

- Low body temperature
- Low-grade chronic fever

## Hair

Changes to hair are common clinical signs of thyroid disease, and can include:

- Hair loss
- Loss of outer edge of eyebrow hair

- Coarse, brittle, strawlike hair
- Thinning, finer hair
- Loss of scalp, underarm, and/or pubic hair

### Skin

Thyroid disease can manifest in a variety of skin-related symptoms that can be clinically observed:

- Dry skin
- Yellowish, jaundiced cast to the skin
- Pallor, paleness of skin, pale lips
- Smooth, young-looking skin
- Loss of skin pigmentation (vitiligo)
- Warm, moist hands and palms
- Hives
- Lesions on the shins (pretibial myxedema or dermopathy)
- Increased acne
- Flushing or ruddiness of face and throat
- Blister-like bumps of the forehead and face (known as milaria bumps)
- Spider veins in face and neck area

### Nails and Hands

Clinical signs of thyroid disease in the nails and hands can include:

- Onycholysis: distal separation from underlying nail bed, also called Plummer's nails
- Soft nails

- Nails that split or break more easily
- Swollen fingertips (acropachy)

## Eyes

Common clinical symptoms include:

- Bulging or protrusion of the eyes
- Red, inflamed, and/or bloodshot eyes
- Dry eyes
- Watery eyes
- Stare in the eyes
- Retraction of upper eyelids, resulting in a wide-eyed look
- Infrequent blinking
- "Lid lag": the upper eyelid doesn't smoothly follow downward movements of the eyes when you look down
- Swelling or puffiness of the eyelids
- Twitching in the eyes
- Uneven motion of upper eyelid
- Uneven pupil dilation in dim light
- Tremor of closed eyelids
- Inflamed cornea

## Weight

Because thyroid affects metabolism significantly, body weight is often an important clinical sign. Changes can include:

- Weight loss, without a change in diet or exercise
- Increased appetite and food intake, without weight gain

- Weight gain, without a change in diet or exercise
- Inability to lose weight, despite reduced intake and/or increased exercise

### Other Clinical Signs

Your practitioner will look for other clinical signs.

- Tremors
- Shaky hands
- Hyperkinetic movements: table drumming, tapping feet, jerky movements
- Low bone density, seen via DEXA scan or X-ray
- Enlarged tonsils
- Enlarged lymph nodes
- A dull facial expression
- Slow movement
- Slow speech
- Hoarseness of voice
- Edema (swelling) of the hands or feet
- Hyperresponsive or overactive reflexes
- Unusually slow reflexes, especially the Achilles reflex

## Thyroid Blood Tests

It's important to understand the thyroid blood tests that may be done as part of your diagnosis. *Note:* In some cases, I've included normal ranges and values associated with different tests, but keep in mind that normal ranges frequently vary from lab to lab, and may be expressed quite differently in various countries. So be sure to get a printout of your lab tests, along with information from the lab and your practitioner on what the normal range is for each test. Most lab reports will provide this along with the results so that you can review where your tests fall according to your particular lab's values.

### Thyroid-Stimulating Hormone (TSH) Test

Most conventional doctors rely on the TSH blood test to diagnose an overactive or underactive thyroid. This test, known variously as the thyroid-stimulating or thyrotropin-stimulating hormone test, measures the amount of TSH in your bloodstream. It is a measure of the pituitary's response to the levels of circulating thyroid hormone.

When the pituitary detects that there isn't enough circulating thyroid hormone, it releases more TSH. TSH is considered a messenger that tells the thyroid to produce more hormone. So a higher-than-normal TSH indicates low thyroid hormone production, or hypothyroidism, and a lower-than-normal TSH indicates hyperthyroidism.

**HYPOTHYROIDISM, UNDERACTIVE THYROID, OR "LOW" THYROID**
- Thyroid gland is not producing enough thyroid hormone.
- Pituitary releases more TSH into blood, telling thyroid, "Make more thyroid hormone."
- TSH goes up ⇒ High TSH

**HYPERTHYROIDISM, OVERACTIVE THYROID, OR "HIGH" THYROID**
- Thyroid gland is producing too much thyroid hormone.
- Pituitary stops releasing TSH into blood, lets levels drop below normal to tell thyroid, "Stop making thyroid hormone."
- TSH goes down ⇒ Low TSH

You'll need to know what the normal values are for the lab that does your bloodwork, because "normal" varies from lab to lab. Normal thyroid ranges are in tremendous flux right now. Throughout the 1980s and 1990s in North America, normal TSH ranged from a low of 0.3 to 0.5 to a high of 5.0 to 6.0. For example, at the lab where they sent my blood when I was first diagnosed in 1995, a TSH of over 5.5 was considered hypothyroid, and under 0.5 was hyperthyroid. Anywhere in between was considered normal, or "euthyroid."

Values below the bottom end of the TSH normal range usually indicate hyperthyroidism. In more severe hyperthyroidism, this level may even be undetectable, or 0. Nonexistent or nearly undetectable TSH levels are also referred to as "suppressed" levels. The lower the TSH, the more suppressed the thyroid is considered to be, and the more hyperthyroid you may be.

Values above the top of the normal range can indicate hypothyroidism, an underactive thyroid. The higher the number, the more hypothyroid or underactive your thyroid is considered to be.

In November 2002, the National Academy of Clinical Biochemistry (NACB), part of the Academy of the American Association for Clinical Chemistry (AACC), issued revised laboratory medicine practice guidelines for the diagnosis and monitoring of thyroid disease. Of particular interest was the following statement in the guidelines:

> [More than] 95% of rigorously screened normal euthyroid volunteers have serum TSH values between 0.4 and 2.5 mIU/L....A serum TSH result between 0.5 and 2.0 mIU/L is generally considered the therapeutic target for a standard L-T4 replacement dose for primary hypothyroidism.

Based on these findings, in January 2003, the American Association of Clinical Endocrinologists (AACE) made an important announcement.

> Until November 2002, doctors had relied on a normal TSH level ranging from 0.5 to 5.0 to diagnose and treat patients with a thyroid disorder who tested outside the boundaries of that range. Now AACE encourages doctors to consider treatment for patients who test outside the boundaries of a narrower margin based on a target TSH level of 0.3 to 3.0. AACE believes the new range will result in proper diagnosis for millions of Americans who suffer from a mild thyroid disorder, but have gone untreated until now.

In the years since the original NACB guidelines were released, many laboratories have yet to adopt these new guidelines, and the medical world is still not in complete agreement about changing the guidelines. This means that for patients who test below 0.5 or above 3.0, whether or not you get diagnosed and treated for a thyroid condition depends on how up-to-date both your laboratory and practitioner are. (See Table 1.)

### Total T4 Test

Total T4, also known as total thyroxine or serum thyroxine, measures the total amount of circulating thyroxine in your blood—the T4 that is bound to protein and the T4 that is unbound. A high value indicates hyperthyroidism; a low value indicates hypothyroidism. But total T4 levels may be artificially high, because pregnancy and estrogen (including the

## TABLE 1. TEST RESULT FOR TSH LEVELS

| | LEVELS Indicating Hyperthyroidism | NORMAL Thyroid Levels | LEVELS Indicating Hypothyroidism |
|---|---|---|---|
| Outdated guidelines* | Below 0.5 | 0.5 to 5.0–6.0 | Above 5.0–6.0 |
| New guidelines as of 2003 | Below 0.3 | 0.3 to 3.0 | Above 3.0 |

*Many laboratories and practitioners still use these outdated guidelines, and all evidence indicates that this will continue.*

estrogen in hormone replacement drugs or birth control pills) raise thyroid-binding globulin, which elevates total T4, even when the levels circulating in your bloodstream are normal. Thyroid hormone that is bound is not available to your body's cells. This is why most practitioners now prefer the free T4 test.

### Free T4 Test

Free T4 measures the unbound thyroxine levels circulating in your bloodstream. Typically, free T4 is elevated in hyperthyroidism and lowered in hypothyroidism. Free T4 is considered a more accurate and reliable test than total T4.

### Total T3 Test

Total T3, also known as total triiodothyronine or serum triiodothyronine, is a measure of bound and unbound T3 in the bloodstream. Typically, the total T3 level is elevated in hyperthyroidism and lowered in hypothyroidism. (Normal range runs approximately 60 to 180 at some labs.)

## Free T3 Test

Free T3 measures unbound triiodothyronine in your bloodstream. Again, this test is considered more accurate than the total T3 test. At some labs, the normal range for free T3 is 2.2 to 4.0.

It is possible to have low or even normal TSH and free T4 levels, but elevated free T3 levels. In that situation, the thyroid is producing very high levels of T3, but normal levels of T4. Measuring free T3 gives more accurate information on which to base a diagnosis, which in this case would confirm hyperthyroidism.

## Thyroglobulin Test

Thyroglobulin, also known as thyroid-binding globulin or TBG, is a protein produced by your thyroid primarily when it is injured or inflamed. A normal thyroid produces low or no thyroglobulin, and so undetectable thyroglobulin levels usually mean normal thyroid function.

Typically, thyroglobulin is elevated in Graves' disease, thyroiditis, and thyroid cancer. It is not elevated, however, if too much thyroid hormone drug is being taken and is causing thyrotoxicosis. This test can, therefore, help differentiate the cause of thyrotoxicosis in some patients.

## T3 Resin Uptake Test

When done with T3 and T4 tests, the T3 resin uptake (T3RU) test is sometimes referred to as the T7 test. This test can help assess whether your thyroid is dysfunctional or hormones are binding in the bloodstream, causing abnormal results. Conditions causing hyperthyroidism typically increase T3RU.

## TRH Test

In the past, the TRH, or thyrotropin-releasing hormone, test was considered a particularly good blood test for detecting subtle underactive thyroid problems. The time involved in the test, however, has made it all but impossible to get from most physicians, and so the test, while a conventional measurement, has fallen out of favor with most endocrinologists. Dr. Raphael Kellman, a New York City–based holistic physician, has called the TRH test the "gold standard for accurately detecting an underactive thyroid." This simple test involves a TSH measurement, followed by an injection of TRH, and then a second TSH test 25 minutes later. If TSH is normal in the first test but elevated in the second test, 10 or above, this points to hypothyroidism. The test is a "stimulation" or "challenge" test, and Dr. Kellman compares diagnosing hypothyroidism to diagnosing diabetes.

In an interview, Dr. Kellman compared the TRH stimulation test to the glucose tolerance test, a challenge test that is used to evaluate glucose response and diagnose diabetes. Like the glucose tolerance test, the TRH test measures not how the thyroid is performing at any given moment, but how the thyroid is performing when it is hormonally challenged—by the presence of the TRH—to produce thyroid hormone. It is a test of thyroid function in action.

"Of the patients I've seen with three or more typical symptoms of underactive thyroid but who have tested 'normal' in standard tests," says Dr. Kellman, "35 to 40 percent actually have underactive thyroids based on the TRH test."

## Reverse T3 Test

When the body is under stress, instead of converting T4 into T3—the active form of thyroid hormone that works at the cellular level—the body makes what is known as reverse T3 (RT3), an inactive form of the T3 hormone, to conserve energy. Some practitioners believe that even when stress is relieved, in some people the body continues to manufacture RT3 instead of active T3. This in turn creates a thyroid problem at the cellular level, yet the TSH lab values may well be normal. The value of RT3 tests is controversial, but these tests have become somewhat more popular with open-minded doctors who are looking to assess a person's full range of thyroid function.

## Thyroid Antibody Blood Tests

Thyroid antibodies are proteins made by the immune system. These proteins may affect you in several ways. They may

- Stimulate your thyroid to work harder
- Block your thyroid's receptors for thyroid hormone or TSH
- Trigger swelling and nodules
- Trigger inflammation, which slowly destroys your thyroid tissue
- Target your eyes or skin, causing Graves' ophthalmopathy or Graves' dermopathy

Typically, antibody testing may be used to help firm up a diagnosis, but the majority of practitioners don't test for or monitor antibodies. Their reasoning is simple: since antibodies are evidence of autoimmune disease, and since they don't really know how to do much of anything to treat the autoimmune aspect of thyroid disease, the antibody levels are of no use to them clinically.

Some practitioners regularly monitor antibody levels, however, because they recognize that these levels can reflect—and even anticipate—changes in the activity and severity of your thyroid dysfunction. In particular, lower antibody levels may indicate improvement, and an absence of antibodies may point to remission in some people.

Following are common tests used to measure the presence of antibodies.

### Thyroid Peroxidase Antibodies Test

One of the most common antibody tests is thyroid peroxidase antibodies test (TPOAb)—also known as antithyroid peroxidase antibodies test. This test is often done as a first step in determining if there is autoimmune thyroid disease. TPO antibodies work against thyroid peroxidase, an enzyme that plays a part in the T4-to-T3 conversion and synthesis process. The presence of TPO antibodies indicates that the thyroid tissue is being destroyed by some disorder. For example, TPO antibodies are detectable in approximately 95 percent of patients with Hashimoto's thyroiditis.

Note: This test is not diagnostic for Graves' disease; only 50 to 85 percent of patients with Graves' disease will test positive for TPO antibodies.

### Antithyroid Microsomal Antibodies Test

Antithyroid microsomal antibodies (antimicrosomal antibodies) are typically elevated with Hashimoto's thyroiditis in 80 percent of cases. However, this test has largely been replaced by the TPOAb test.

### Thyroglobulin Antibodies Test

About 60 percent of patients with Hashimoto's disease and 30 percent of patients with Graves' disease test positive for thyroglobulin antibodies (also called antithyroglobulin antibodies). Patients with Graves' disease who have high levels of thyroglobulin antibodies are more likely to become hypothyroid.

## Thyroid Receptor Antibodies Test

Thyroid receptor antibodies (TRAb) are seen in most patients with a history of Graves' disease. There are different kinds of TRAb, including:

- Stimulatory, in which case they cause hyperthyroidism (TSH-stimulating antibodies [TSAb])
- Blocking, in which case they prevent TSH from binding to the cell receptor and cause hypothyroidism (TSH receptor blocking antibodies [TBAb/TSBAb])
- Binding, in which case they interfere with the activity of TSH at the cell receptor

Patients with Graves' disease tend to test positive for stimulatory TSAb, and patients with Hashimoto's disease tend to test positive for blocking TBAb.

## Test for Thyroid-Stimulating Immunoglobulin

Thyroid-stimulating immunoglobulin (TSI) can be detected in 75 to 90 percent of Graves' disease patients. Its presence is considered diagnostic for Graves' disease: the higher the levels, the more active the Graves' disease. The absence of these antibodies does not mean that you don't have Graves' disease, however.

Monitoring TSI levels may help predict a relapse of Graves' disease, and lower TSI levels can indicate that treatment is working.

TSI monitoring is particularly important during pregnancy. Elevated levels during pregnancy—particularly in early pregnancy and during the third trimester—are a risk factor for fetal or neonatal thyroid dysfunction, because the mother's antibodies can transfer to an unborn baby via the placenta, making a baby hyperthyroid in utero or at birth. Research has shown that as many as 10 percent of pregnant women with elevated TSI levels deliver hyperthyroid babies.

Some people with autoimmune hypothyroidism also have TSI, and this can cause periodic transient hyperthyroid episodes.

## Thyroid Imaging Tests

A variety of imaging and evaluation tests are used to make a more conclusive diagnosis.

### Radioactive Iodine Uptake (RAI-U)

Radioactive iodine uptake (RAI-U) is a nuclear scan test that is done to help differentiate between Graves' disease, toxic multinodular goiter, and thyroiditis. A small dose of radioactive iodine 123 is administered as a pill. Several hours later, the amount of iodine in the system is measured, often accompanied by an X-ray that views how much iodine is concentrated in the thyroid.

Intake of high amounts of iodine in the diet can interfere with the test results, so your doctor will typically recommend that you fast before the test. Find out from your doctor how long you should fast. Be sure to tell your doctor about any medications or supplements you are taking, particularly those that contain iodine, such as multivitamins, kelp, bladderwrack, and seaweed.

Also keep in mind that if you've had medical tests that used iodine contrast dyes, this may skew your RAI-U results for weeks or months and make the test results less accurate. Be sure to mention any of these tests to your doctor before having RAI-U.

An overactive thyroid usually takes up higher amounts of iodine than normal, and that uptake is visible in the X-ray. A thyroid that takes up iodine is considered "hot"—overactive— as opposed to a "cold," or underactive, thyroid.

In Graves' disease, RAI-U is elevated, and the entire gland becomes hot. (By contrast, in Hashimoto's thyroiditis the uptake is usually low, with patchy hot spots in the gland.)

RAI-U can show hot or cold thyroid nodules. If you are hyperthyroid because of a nodule, and not Graves' disease, the nodule will show up as hot and the rest of your thyroid will be cold. Hot nodules may overproduce thyroid hormone, but they are rarely cancerous. An estimated 10 to 20 percent of cold nodules are cancerous, however.

Almost all forms of hyperthyroidism show as higher uptake. In rare cases, you can have a cold scan with low uptake but still be hyperthyroid. That situation happens typically only if you are thyrotoxic from overexposure to thyroid hormone.

Lab work takes time. Many doctors prefer the RAI-U test because they can do it in their own office and get results quickly. (They can also charge for it.) Some practitioners believe that this test is not as accurate or as safe as blood tests in diagnosing Graves' disease.

*Note:* Radioactive iodine 131 (I-31) is used for ablation of the thyroid and for cancer treatment. RAI-U uses I-123, which gives off a very low level of radiation. It has a very short half-life, approximately 13 hours, so an accurate RAI-U scan can be performed as soon as 20 minutes after an intravenous administration, or from 1 to 24 hours after taking it orally. With a typical oral dose of 100 to 300 millicuries, an accurate scan can be done after 6 hours. Technetium 99M is sometimes used in women who are breastfeeding, because its half-life is 6 hours. The radioactivity dissipates quickly and a nursing mother could get back to breastfeeding her infant more quickly.

Because this test involves radioactivity, it is not performed on pregnant women under any circumstances.

### Computed Tomography

Computed tomography, known as CT scan or "cat scan," is a specialized type of X-ray that is used infrequently to evaluate the thyroid. A CT scan cannot detect small nodules, but it can diagnose a goiter or larger nodules.

### Magnetic Resonance Imaging

Magnetic resonance imaging (MRI) is done when the size and shape of the thyroid needs to be evaluated. MRI can't tell anything about how your thyroid is functioning—whether it is hyperthyroid or hypothyroid—but it can detect enlargement, and may be used in conjunction with blood tests. It is sometimes preferable to X-rays or CT scans because it doesn't require any injection of contrast dye, and doesn't require radiation.

### Orbital CT Scan or MRI

CT scan or MRI of the eye orbit is sometimes done to diagnose Graves' ophthalmopathy if a patient has Graves' disease antibodies but normal thyroid hormone levels.

## Thyroid Ultrasound

Ultrasound of the thyroid is done to evaluate nodules, lumps, and enlargement of the gland. Ultrasound can also determine whether a nodule is a fluid-filled cyst or a mass of solid tissue. It cannot determine whether a nodule or lump is benign or malignant, however.

In Graves' disease, the thyroid is usually enlarged. A reduction in the size of the thyroid is one of the first signs that you are responding to treatment. If you are on antithyroid drugs, your doctor may use ultrasound to monitor the success of your treatment.

## Needle Biopsy or Fine Needle Aspiration

This technique helps to evaluate lumps or cold nodules. In a needle biopsy, a thin needle is inserted directly into the lump and some cells are withdrawn and evaluated. In some cases, ultrasound is used to help guide the needle into the correct position. Pathology assessment of the cells can often reveal Hashimoto's thyroiditis, as well as cancerous cells. Definitive information is available in approximately 75 percent of nodules biopsied.

## Other Blood Tests

A physician may do other bloodwork to rule out thyroid disease or identify related conditions that may raise the suspicion of a thyroid condition.

Other blood test results that may be pointing to (but are not conclusively diagnostic of) thyroid conditions include:

- High sedimentation ("sed" rate)
- Abnormal (high or low) cholesterol
- Abnormal (high or low) triglycerides
- Abnormal (high or low) iron or ferritin
- Elevated serum calcium
- Elevated alkaline phosphatase
- Elevated sex hormone–binding globulin levels
- Elevated blood sugar or poor glucose tolerance
- Elevated hemoglobin A1C
- Elevated bilirubin
- Elevated aminotransferases
- Decreased free testosterone levels
- Elevated C-reactive protein levels
- Elevated homocysteine levels

## Diagnosing Thyroid Disorders

These are the usual tests performed on most patients. Radioactive scans are not generally performed on pregnant or breast-feeding women. This is discussed in more detail in Chapter 7.

### *Hypothyroidism*

Conventional doctors will typically start with a thyroid-stimulating hormone (TSH) blood test. As discussed previously, levels above 3.0 to 6.0 indicate hypothroidism (see Table 1 on page 48).

*Note:* Some practitioners believe that the optimal TSH level for becoming pregnant and maintaining the pregnancy is actually between 1.0 and 2.0, and they would consider a TSH of 2.0 to 3.0 to be slightly elevated and possibly deserving of thyroid hormone replacement treatment.

Total and free T4 and T3 tests are also commonly used to help diagnose hypothyroidism. Low levels on any of these tests, in conjunction with elevated TSH levels, may indicate hypothyroidism.

## Hashimoto's Thyroiditis

Hashimoto's thyroiditis is the autoimmune disease that is the most common cause of hypothyroidism. The characteristic Hashimoto's thyroiditis patient would have high TSH values and, usually, low T3 and T4 thyroid hormone levels. However, the greatest distinguishing feature for Hashimoto's is a high concentration of thyroid autoantibodies—anti-TPO antibodies in particular. Some patients have elevations in antibody levels for months, or even years, before the TSH level becomes elevated.

## Hyperthyroidism

As with hypothyroidism, doctors will typically begin with a TSH blood test. As discussed prevously, levels below 0.3 to 0.5 indicate hyperthyroidism (see Table 1 on page 48).

Total and free T3 and T4 tests are also used to help diagnose hyperthyroidism. High levels on any of these tests, along with a low TSH, may indicate hyperthyroidism.

## Graves' Disease

The thyroid-stimulating antibodies (TSAb) or thyroid-stimulating immunoglobulin (TSI) in your blood may also be measured to diagnose Graves' disease, the autoimmune condition that frequently causes hyperthyroidism.

A radioactive scan of the thyroid, using I-123 taken by mouth, may also be taken to see if the thyroid gland is overactive. Overactivity of the thyroid gland is a hallmark of Graves' disease.

### Goiter

Several steps can be involved in diagnosing goiter.

- Examining and observing your neck for enlargement
- A blood test to determine if your thyroid is producing irregular amounts of thyroid hormone
- Antibodies testing, to confirm that autoimmune disease may be the cause of your goiter
- An ultrasound test to evaluate the degree of the enlargement
- A radioactive isotope thyroid scan to produce an image of the thyroid and provide visual information about the nature of the thyroid enlargement.

### Thyroid Nodules

Nodules are usually evaluated by:

- A blood test, to determine whether the nodules are producing thyroid hormone
- A radioactive thyroid scan, which looks at the reaction of the nodule to small amounts of radioactive material
- An ultrasound of the thyroid, to determine whether the nodule is solid or fluid-filled
- A fine-needle aspiration or needle biopsy of the nodules, to evaluate whether they may be cancerous.

## Thyroid Cancer

The main diagnostic procedure for suspected thyroid cancer is typically a fine-needle aspiration (FNA) of the thyroid nodule. Fluid and cells are removed from various parts of all nodules that can be felt, and these samples are then evaluated. Sometimes FNA tests are done with an ultrasound machine to help guide the needle into nodules that are too small to be felt. Between 60 percent and 80 percent of FNA tests show that the nodule is benign. About 1 of 20 (5 percent) FNA tests reveals cancer. The remainder of cases are classified as "suspicious," and frequently a surgical biopsy is ordered to rule out or diagnose cancer.

A radioactive thyroid scan may be done to identify if the nodules are cold, which means they have a greater potential to be cancerous.

# Alternative Testing and Self-Testing

Symptoms of a thyroid condition should not be viewed casually, and you must always see a health care professional as soon as possible for evaluation and diagnosis. It can be helpful, however, to use self-checks and alternative testing as a way to stay on top of your health, to get tests that HMOs and insurance companies may deny coverage for, or to benefit from early detection.

## The Thyroid Neck Check

One simple at-home self-test that can potentially detect some thyroid abnormalities is a thyroid neck check. To take this test, hold a mirror so that you can see your thyroid area—the neck area just below the Adam's apple and above the collarbone. Tip your head back, while keeping this view of your neck and thyroid area in your mirror. Take a drink of water and swallow. As you swallow, look at your neck. Watch carefully for any bulges, enlargement, protrusions, or unusual appearances in this area. Repeat this process several times. If you see anything that appears unusual, see your doctor right away. You may have a goiter (an enlarged thyroid) or a thyroid nodule, and your thyroid should be evaluated. Be sure you don't get your Adam's apple confused with your thyroid gland. The Adam's apple is at the front of your neck; the thyroid is farther down, and closer to your collarbone. Remember that this test is by no means conclusive and cannot rule out thyroid abnormalities. It's just helpful to identify a particularly enlarged thyroid or masses in the thyroid that warrant evaluation.

### Basal Body Temperature Test

Thyroid hormones have a direct effect on the basal, or resting, metabolic rate. And while hypothermia, or lowered body temperature, is a known and medically accepted symptom of hypothyroidism, the use of body temperature as a diagnostic tool is more controversial. The late Broda Barnes, M.D., made the public more widely aware of the use of axillary (underarm) basal body temperature (BBT) as a symptom and diagnostic tool for hypothyroidism. It is a diagnostic and monitoring method still used by some alternative practitioners.

To measure your BBT, use an oral thermometer or a special BBT thermometer available at some pharmacies. If you are using a glass thermometer, shake it down before you go to bed and leave it within easy reach. As soon as you wake up, and with minimal movement, put the thermometer in your armpit, next to the skin, and leave it for 10 minutes. Record the readings for three to five consecutive days. Women should not use this test during the first four days of their period, but can begin on day 5. Record your results in Table 2.

## TABLE 2. BASAL BODY TEMPERATURE TEST RESULTS

| Day 1 | Day 2 | Day 3 | Day 4 | Day 5 | Day 6 | Day 7 | Day 8 | Day 9 | Day 10 |
|-------|-------|-------|-------|-------|-------|-------|-------|-------|--------|
|       |       |       |       |       |       |       |       |       |        |

Average BBT: Days 1–5 ___        Days 6–10 ___        Days 1–10 ___

If your average BBT is below 97.6 Fahrenheit, some alternative practitioners would consider a diagnosis of an underfunctioning thyroid or insufficient thyroid hormone replacement. An average BBT between 97.8 and 98.2 is considered normal. Temperatures from 97.6 to 98.0 degrees Fahrenheit are considered evidence of possible hypothyroidism, and temperatures less than 97.6 degrees can be even more indicative of hypothyroidism. Some practitioners, however, consider any temperature under 98 degrees to be indicative of hypothyroidism.

Use of basal body temperature is controversial, however, and even those practitioners who use the test caution that it should be part of an overall approach. According to holistic thyroid expert and author Dr. Richard Shames:

> For those who have already been diagnosed with hypothyroidism, the basal temperature test is an additional piece of observational measurement that helps determine whether a person is on the right medicine and/or the right dose, along with considering the response to medication, physical signs (especially ankle reflexes and skin temperature), and blood test results. Temperature testing, however, is not infallible,

and—like any other test—should never be used alone to rule in or rule out a thyroid condition, or to dictate therapy. This is simply a good piece of information that should be used wisely.

## Iodine Skin Test

Some practitioners and alternative health resources recommend testing for iodine skin absorption: put a patch of iodine on the skin of the arm; see if it disappears, and if so, how quickly. This is a very controversial test, and even innovative alternative practitioners have serious doubts about the validity of this test. Retired thyroid expert Dr. David Derry had this to say in an interview.

> The "test" of putting iodine on the skin to watch how fast it disappears is not an indicator of anything. The iodine disappearance rate is unrelated to thyroid disease or even iodine content of the body. When iodine is applied to the skin in almost any form, 50% evaporates into the air within 2 hours and between 75 and 80 percent evaporates into the air within 24 hours.

## Order Your Own Laboratory Tests

Some options for blood testing do not require a doctor and prescription. HealthCheckUSA offers three different test options: a standard TSH test; the Comprehensive Thyroid Profile, which includes T3 uptake, T4 total, T7, and TSH tests; and the Comprehensive Thyroid Profile II, which includes free T3 (triiodothyronine), free T4 (thyroxine), and TSH tests. The tests are extremely affordable, HealthCheckUSA doctors sign off on blood work requests, you have the blood drawn at a designated lab in your area, and you receive the results directly, online or by mail. You can order tests by calling 1–800–929–2044 or by visiting the website at http://www. thyroidbreakthrough.com

### Saliva Testing

Saliva testing is another means of thyroid testing that some alternative practitioners use as an adjunct to blood tests. But I've yet to talk to a holistic practitioner who regularly uses saliva testing for diagnosing or managing hypothyroidism on a large patient population. Even those practitioners who rely on saliva testing to evaluate adrenal function or levels of hormones such as cortisol and progesterone feel that saliva testing for thyroid function is less reliable.

### Urinary Testing

Some doctors who follow the approaches to diagnosis and treatment outlined by the late Dr. Broda Barnes use a 24-hour urine collection test to evaluate for hypothyroidism. The test, which is evaluated by a laboratory in Belgium, measures the levels of T3 and T4 in 24-hour urine samples. This is a controversial test; some practitioners find it useful, and others say it's unproven.

## Diagnosis Controversies

It's important to note that there is a major controversy between those practitioners who believe that blood tests must be abnormal in order to diagnose thyroid disease and justify treatment and those practitioners who feel that blood tests are only a small part of the picture. Dr. Steven Hotze argues that TSH tests are not the reliable diagnostic tools some physicians believe them to be. "Hypothyroidism is a clinical diagnosis," says Hotze. "TSH doesn't measure intracellular thyroid, and it's not even a measure of thyroid hormone itself, it's a secondary test."

Hotze believes in using clinical history and evaluation and a therapeutic trial of thyroid hormone with patients who fit the classic thyroid symptoms. Blood tests are done, but only to provide a baseline upon which to evaluate changes, not as a diagnostic arbiter. As Dr. Hotze says, "If it's all just about the TSH test, why even see the patient? Why not give them a number, draw blood, and treat the blood test?"

This is in contrast to the conventional approach. Most endocrinologists believe that unless blood tests show clear and incontrovertible evidence of thyroid dysfunction, even a family and personal history and symptoms and clinical signs, such as goiter, weight gain, slow reflexes, and hair loss, for example, are not enough evidence upon which to make a diagnosis. According to the American Association of Clinical Endocrinologists,

> Treating patients with *any* type of thyroid hormone solely because they have symptoms that are commonly associated with hypothyroidism is potentially hazardous. Such symptoms are also very common in the general population, most of whom do *not* have hypothyroidism and will *not* experience any sustained improvement in their symptoms with thyroid hormone therapy. A scientifically-based diagnosis of hypothyroidism must be made before initiating therapy.

Interestingly, it has been almost four years since the AACE issued revised standards for TSH levels (see page 47). Yet American doctors and laboratories have yet to adopt these standards. As a result, as many as 30 million thyroid patients are excluded from proper diagnosis and treatment.

It's unlikely that the controversies surrounding diagnosis and treatment will be settled anytime soon.

In the meantime, you may wish to patronize those physicians and practitioners who are willing to treat you as a whole person—who will take into account your medical history, symptoms, and clinical signs as part of their decision making—rather than relying solely on the results of blood tests.

# Chapter 4

# Thyroid Treatment

One of the most sublime experiences we can ever have is to wake up feeling healthy after we have been sick.

—Rabbi Harold Kushner

The end result for most thyroid patients is hypothyroidism—an underactive thyroid condition that requires thyroid hormone replacement for life.

With Hashimoto's disease, the thyroid typically burns itself out over time, becoming less able to produce thyroid hormone and leaving most patients hypothyroid.

With Graves' disease and hyperthyroidism, most doctors ablate the thyroid with radioactive iodine, which leaves patients without a functional thyroid. The patient starts out with an overactive gland and ends up hypothyroid. Many doctors do not explain this fully to patients when they recommend this treatment.

With thyroid nodules and goiter, surgery may be performed to remove all or part of the thyroid. The end result is frequently hypothyroidism.

And for thyroid cancer, almost all patients have their thyroid removed entirely, leaving them completely hypothyroid and reliant on thyroid hormone replacement.

## Optimizing Your Treatment

Because thyroid hormone replacement may be the most fundamental aspect of your thyroid treatment, it's important to ensure that your treatment is optimal. Here are some important questions to address.

### *Are You on the Right Brand of Levothyroxine?*

Most people start out taking levothyroxine, a synthetic form of the T4 hormone thyroxine. But some people simply do not feel well on some brands of levothyroxine, and sometimes changing brands seems to help. There are a number of FDA-approved brands available (Synthroid, Levoxyl, Levothroid, and others). You may wish to discuss a change with your physician. Do stick with a brand name, however, and not a generic, to ensure consistency. (Every time you refill a generic prescription, you may get a different manufacturer's product.)

### *Do You Need to Add T3?*

Some people do not feel their best without the addition of the active thyroid hormone T3. Usually, the body converts T4 to T3, but nutritional deficiencies, toxins, and a variety of other physiological factors may prevent the body from accomplishing that conversion process properly, leaving you deficient in this most important thyroid hormone. While the matter is still under study, some physicians believe that supplemental T3 may optimize thyroid treatment for some patients. They may add T3 in one of several ways:

- Levothyroxine treatment plus the prescription T3 drug Cytomel.
- Compounded time-released T3 in addition to levothyroxine
- Combination synthetic drug Thyrolar, which includes both T4 and T3
- Natural desiccated thyroid, which also includes a full array of natural thyroid hormones, including T3

Check with your physician about whether supplemental T3 might be a help for you.

### Would Natural Thyroid Help?

Some practitioners believe that certain patients simply do best on natural desiccated thyroid, which is derived from the thyroid gland of pigs. These products, including Armour, Biotech, and Nature-throid, are prescription thyroid drugs that have been in use for over 100 years. Alternative practioners believe that these drugs, which provide T4, T3, T2, T1, and other thyroid hormones and nutritional elements, more closely resemble human thyroid hormone than synthetics, and report that their patients feel better on these drugs. Many conventional physicians feel that these drugs are out of date and won't prescribe them, so you may need to find an open-minded doctor, or a holistic or alternative physician, to prescribe them.

Diana was suffering with hypothyroidism after pregnancy, with constant bleeding and other hormonal symptoms, until her gynecologist decided to take her off Synthroid and try Armour.

> That decision was the turning point in my life. That decision
> stopped my suicidal thoughts, my thoughts of worthlessness
> and wanting to end it all. I am becoming more well day-by-
> day. My periods are now back to the way they were *before* I
> ever became pregnant, lasting only five days, my hair is shiny
> and soft without the addition of anything after washing, my
> skin has moisture in it again, and I feel *good*! All it took on her
> [gynecologist's] part was logical thinking. She did not suggest
> the invasive surgeries that the other doctors threw at me and
> she listened when I told her I did not feel well.

## Are You at the Optimal Dosage of TSH?

Each laboratory determines its own normal range for TSH levels, but where you personally feel best will vary. A study reported in the *Journal of Clinical Endocrinology and Metabolism* found that the mean TSH level for people who don't have a thyroid condition is 1.5, and the American Association of Clinical Endocrinologists has set the normal range for TSH levels at 0.3 to 3.0. Nevertheless, many practitioners and labs are still using the outdated 0.5 to 5.0 range, leaving millions of people undiagnosed, untreated, and at risk of a host of reproductive problems.

If your TSH is on the higher end of normal for you, you may have PMS, irregular periods, fertility problems, or a more difficult menopause. Check your most recent blood test results and consult with your physician about whether a slight reduction in your TSH levels would be better for your health.

One other little-known issue for thyroid patients is the seasonal variation in thyroid function. A number of studies show that TSH naturally rises during the colder months and drops to low normal or even hyperthyroid levels in the warmest months. Some doctors adjust for this by prescribing slightly increased dosages during the colder months, and reducing the dosage during warm periods. Most, doctors are not aware of this seasonal fluctuation, however, leaving patients to suffer from worsening hypothyroidism symptoms during colder months. This seasonal fluctuation becomes more pronounced in older people and in particularly cold climates. Twice-yearly tests, at minimum during winter and summer months, can identify these fluctuations and guide any seasonal dosage modifications needed.

When Tara started having perimenopausal symptoms, her doctors gave her estrogen and progesterone, but she did not feel well.

I found out later by checking out my earlier thyroid lab tests that I was not being given enough thyroid medication. The doctor I had at this time tested me for various things, and had me try various supplements, but she somehow never noticed my thyroid levels were in the low range. I went to six more doctors and endocardiologists after her and none helped. I saw one endo who said, "Nothing is wrong with you. It doesn't matter that you feel lousy." I saw another doctor who laughed and said, "You are the healthiest person I have seen all week." Another, who felt low estrogen was the problem, gave me so much estrogen I wound up in the hospital with a D and C for bleeding problems. Luckily a couple of girlfriends kept encouraging me to not give up and continue to try new doctors. Finally one of them "got it." He literally gave me back my life!

## Are You Taking Your Medication Properly?

There are a number of guidelines on how to take thyroid hormone properly, to ensure that you are absorbing the drug and receiving the maximum possible benefit.

- Don't take your thyroid hormone replacement drug within four hours of taking calcium supplements, calcium-fortified juice, or antacids such as Tums or Mylanta, which also contain calcium. Calcium can delay or reduce the absorption of your thyroid hormone.
- Don't take thyroid hormone replacement drugs within four hours of taking any supplements that contain iron, including prenatal vitamins, which are usually high in iron.
- Try to take your thyroid hormone around the same time each day. For best results, maximum absorption, and minimum interference from food, fiber, and supplements, doctors recommend taking it in the morning on an empty stomach, about an hour before eating.
- If you need to take your thyroid hormone with food, be consistent and *always* take it with food. Don't switch back and forth.
- If you start or stop a high-fiber diet while you are on thyroid hormone, have your thyroid function retested around six to eight weeks after your dietary change. High-fiber diets can change the speed of thyroid drug

absorption, and you may require a dosage adjustment. You should also be consistent about your daily fiber intake. Don't have 10 grams one day, 30 grams the next day, and so on, or you risk erratic absorption.

- If you are taking Levoxyl, be sure to take the drug with enough water and swallow the pill quickly. The pill dissolves rapidly; if it dissolves in your mouth, not your stomach, you risk not absorbing all of the active ingredients.

## Is Optimizing Treatment Really Important?

Thyroid experts Drs. Richard and Karilee Shames, emphasize the critical importance of optimizing thryoid treatment.

A lack of proper thyroid hormone levels has been implicated in everything from bad PMS to irregular cycles, low libido, infertility, miscarriage, endometriosis, polycystic ovary, uterine fibroids, dysfunctional bleeding, severe menopause, and osteoporosis. With a long list of possible gynecological problems such as this, you are well advised to optimize your thyroid function as much as possible. Perhaps even more important is for the person who is already diagnosed and being treated for low thyroid to make sure that your treatment protocol is optimal. In my coaching practice, where I speak with women from all over the country, I frequently find someone who is experiencing uncomfortable symptoms of female hormone imbalance due to an inadequate dose of thyroid medicine. Often these symptoms completely disappear without further female hormone intervention simply through the proper thyroid care alone. Keep in mind there are at least five (5) different kinds of synthetic thyroid, and five (5) different kinds of natural thyroid, in addition to Armour. Sometimes it's not just the dose of your medicine, it's the type or brand—and don't forget that many women need a mix of thyroids rather than just one type.

## Nutrition and Supplements for Thyroid Function

You'll also want to make sure that you are getting proper nutritional supplements to help support your thyroid.

### Multivitamins

A high-potency multivitamin is essential for thyroid patients. Look for one that has high amounts of vitamins B, C, and E and a good range of minerals. One that I particularly like is Dr. Jacob Teitelbaum's formulation known as Daily Energy Enfusion. Dr. Teitelbaum's formula does contain some iodine, however, so you may want to slightly reduce your daily dosage if you are iodine-sensitive. The vitamin comes as a flavorful powdered drink along with one vitamin B capsule; this replaces more than 30 vitamins and supplement pills each day. Dr. Teitelbaum's formula does not include iron or calcium, so it can be taken at the same time as thyroid pills.

### Probiotics

Probiotics are supplements that contain live bacteria—the "good" bacteria found in fermented foods such as miso and dairy products such as yogurt and some cheeses—that we are meant to have in sufficient quantities in our intestinal system. One of the more well-known probiotics is acidophilus, the live culture found in yogurt.

According to a report in the *European Journal of Clinical Nutrition*, the probiotic known as bifidobacterium lactis HN019 boosts the activity of various disease-killing immune system cells in healthy adults. Probiotics help proper digestive functioning, which enhances the immune system. They also kill off harmful bacteria, having an antibiotic effect by fighting off various types of infection. But the concentration of live cultures in yogurt is not high enough to get a substantial effect, so a probiotic supplement is your best option. Some probiotic supplements can be expensive and require refrigeration, but I recommend a patented formula from Enzymatic Therapies, called Acidophilus Pearls. This tiny pearl-shaped supplement contains a guaranteed level of live bacteria in the millions, is very inexpensive, and requires no refrigeration.

### Zinc

Zinc is important for thyroid hormone production and conversion, and 15 to 25 mg of zinc a day can help ensure optimum zinc delivery to the thyroid. Zinc, along with selenium, can also help prevent the decline of T3 when you are on a lower-calorie diet.

### Selenium

Research has shown that selenium is an important mineral for thyroid function. The conversion of T4 to T3 is in part controlled by selenium. Selenium activates an enzyme responsible for controlling thyroid function by the conversion of T4 to T3. Stress and injury also appear to make the body particularly thyroid-responsive and selenium-deficient. Supplemental selenium also appears to offset the effect of high iodine intake on thyroid function. A 1997 study suggested that high intake of iodine when selenium is deficient may cause thyroid damage. Selenium supplementation has also been shown to reduce inflammation and antibody levels in patients with autoimmune thyroiditis. Too much selenium can be dangerous, so multivitamin and additional supplementation should not exceed 400 mcg per day.

## L-Tyrosine

L-tyrosine is a known precursor to thyroid hormone, and low levels can make it difficult for the thyroid to function properly. It is a common component of many thyroid support supplements that combine several supplements into one capsule. Tyrosine supplements at the level of 85 to 170 mg a day may be a help to the thyroid.

## Z-Guggulsterone

Z-guggulsterone, also known as guggul, a component derived from the plant commiphora mukul, has been used in Ayurvedic medicine as an anti-inflammatory, antiobesity, thyroid-stimulating, and cholesterol-lowering agent. Guggul is considered particularly important for the prevention of a sluggish metabolism. Studies have shown that it can increase the thyroid's ability to take up the enzymes it needs for effective hormone conversion, and also increase the oxygen uptake in muscles. Some people find that guggul is overstimulating, so you need to be careful using this supplement.

## Essential Fatty Acids

Essential fatty acids (EFAs) cannot be produced in the body, so you must get them through diet or supplements. The key essential fatty acids include:

- Omega-3 fatty acids: alpha linolenic acid (ALA), eicosapentaenoic acid (EPA), and docosahexaenoic acid (DHA). These are found in fresh fish from the deep ocean (mackerel, tuna, herring, flounder, sardines, salmon, rainbow trout, bass), as well as in linseed oil, flaxseeds and flaxseed oil, black currant and pumpkin seeds, cod liver oil, shrimp, oysters, leafy greens, soybeans, walnuts, wheat germ, fresh sea vegetables, and fish oil. Usually, your body can convert ALA into EPA, and then into DHA.
- Omega-6 fatty acids: linoleic acid and gamma-linolenic acid (GLA). These are found in breast milk, sesame, safflower, cotton, and sunflower seeds and oil, corn and corn oil, soybeans, and raw nuts, legumes, leafy greens, black currant seeds, evening primrose oil, borage oil, spirulina, soybeans, and lecithin. Linoleic acid in omega-6 can be converted into GLA.

According to Dr. Udo Erasmus, author of *Fats That Heal, Fats That Kill*, imbalances and deficiencies in EFAs are the cause, a trigger, or a contributing factor in many diseases and conditions. Addressing those deficiencies through proper foods, or use of healthy oils can have huge implications for health. He believes that EFAs are critical to thyroid function for three reasons: They are required for the integrity of the structure of every membrane of every cell. They increase energy levels in the cell. And there is some evidence that essential fatty acids, especially omega-3s, improve the body's ability to detect and respond to thyroid hormone effectively.

Dr. Erasmus also points to the role that EFAs play in preventing and reducing inflammation. In particular, essential fatty acids make hormone-like eicosanoids that regulate immune and inflammatory responses, and omega-3s in particular have anti-inflammatory effects that can slow autoimmune damage. Inflammation of the thyroid—known as goiter—is central to many cases of autoimmune thyroid disease, and inflammation is seen in almost all autoimmune diseases.

Dr. Erasmus believes that if proteins are the juice, fats are the insulators, not just of nerves but of cells and membranes. Protein reactions lead to inflammation, allergies, and autoimmune disease. Essential fatty acids seem to help prevent proteins from becoming hyperactive, and thereby triggering these various immune reactions.

You can add EFAs to your diet by increasing foods rich in these substances and by taking supplements.

- Omega-3 fish oil supplements: Go for a decent-tasting oil or a "burpless" capsule. Enzymatic Therapies' Eskimo Oil is my favorite.
- Omega-3 flaxseeds and flaxseed oil: You can add flaxseed oils to meals, either in the oil form or as capsules. Some people like to make salad dressing out of the oil or add it to soups. Taking flaxseed oil with each meal helps slow down digestion and modulate blood sugar fluctuations (which helps with insulin levels).
- Omega-6 evening primrose oil or borage oil: These are usually taken as supplements. GLA is thought to help activate brown fat—an energy-burning, heat-generating "good" type of fat—which can boost the metabolic efficiency.

If you want to include a healthy balance of EFAs, think about a product that includes a balance of oils, such Dr. Erasmus's Udo's Oil products.

## Some Cautions

### Watch Goitrogens

Goitrogens are products and foods that promote the formation of goiters. They can act like antithyroid drugs by disabling the thyroid and causing hypothyroidism. Specifically, goitrogens inhibit the body's ability to use iodine, block the process by which iodine becomes T3 and T4, inhibit the actual secretion of thyroid hormone, and disrupt the peripheral conversion of T4 to T3.

If you are hypothyroid due to thyroidectomy, you don't have to be particularly concerned about goitrogens. If you still have a thyroid, however, you need to be careful not to eat uncooked goitrogens in large quantities. The enzymes involved in the formation of goitrogenic materials in plants can be partially destroyed by cooking. Eating moderate amounts of goitrogenic foods, raw or cooked, is probably not a problem for most people.

The following is a list of some of the more common and potent goitrogens:

| | |
|---|---|
| African cassava | Kohlrabi |
| Babassu (palm-tree nut found in Brazil and Africa) | Millet |
| | Mustard |
| Broccoli | Radishes |
| Brussels sprouts | Rutabaga |
| Cabbage | Soy products |
| Cauliflower | Turnips |
| Kale | Watercress |

## Reduce Toxic Exposure

When it comes to fluoride, it's not often known that it has been used as a medication for the treatment of *hyperthyroidism*—meaning that it has the ability to suppress thyroid function. In one study, it was shown that 2.3 to 4.5 mg of fluoride per day was a successful treatment for hyperthyroidism. In areas where water is fluoridated, typical fluoride intake ranges from 1.6 to 6.6 mg/day, which in some cases exceeds the dosage used for medical treatment of hyperthyroidism. What you can do? Drink bottled water that is not fluoridated. Use a fluoride-free toothpaste. And do not get dental fluoride treatments at the dentist. These treatments have not been clearly demonstrated to reduce or prevent cavities in adults.

Perchlorate, a chemical that is known to disrupt thyroid function and cause other health problems, is increasingly the focus of public and government attention. The U.S. water supply, especially in the West, has become contaminated with perchlorate. Produce may also have residues of perchlorate from fertilizers and water. Foods grown with perchlorate-tainted fertilizers can be contaminated. There's not much you can do to avoid eating such produce except to grow your own food and water it with perchlorate-free water. Well water should be tested for perchlorate, and if you live in an area near a current or former facility for rockets, explosives, or fireworks production, you should also consider having your water tested. Most important, become aware of the issues and monitor the status of perchlorate legislation by visiting the comprehensive site, http://www.perchlorate.org.

Some practitioners believe that mercury is toxic to the immune system and, in particular, the thyroid. Mercury exposure comes not only through dental fillings, but also by eating some types of fish, which may contain high levels of mercury. Mercury levels can be tested by a holistic physician or nutritionist, using hair analysis for metals and minerals. If you have excessive levels of mercury, some experts recommend chelation—the process of helping the body excrete excess metals and minerals. This can be done through IV infusion or herbal supplements. In some cases, practitioners recommend removing mercury fillings and replacing them with composite materials that contain no mercury. This is controversial, because it can be very expensive. Some patients have reported that their thyroid problems and other symptoms were greatly relieved with removal of mercury fillings.

## Treat Infections

Infection with food-borne bacteria may also be a trigger for some thyroid problems. *Yersinia enterocolitica*, for example, has been associated with production and elevated levels of thyroid antibodies, a sign of autoimmune thyroid disease.

A specialized analysis by the Great Smokies Diagnostics Laboratory—typically ordered by your physician—can help detect intestinal bacterial overgrowth that may be contributing to underlying immune system problems and fueling the thyroid condition. These are treated with antibiotics, or, if you are working with a more holistic practitioner, diet, nutritional supplements, and herbs that function in an antibiotic-like capacity.

## Watch Out for Soy

There is much debate and controversy regarding the pros and cons of soy. But there is increasing agreement that overconsumption of isoflavone-intensive soy products may pose more prob-

lems than benefits, especially when it comes to women's reproductive health. It's important to understand that the popularity
of soy as a plant estrogen, or phytoestrogen, means that soy acts
as a weak hormone, operating like estrogen in the body.

The isoflavones in soy belong to the flavonoid chemical
family, and flavonoids are considered endocrine disrupters—
plants that act as hormones, disrupting the endocrine system.
At high levels, soy also has antithyroid properties. Flavonoids
typically act against the thyroid by inhibition of thyroid peroxidase (TPO), which disturbs proper thyroid function. Soy
also fits into the body's estrogen-receptor and thyroid-receptor
sites, where it can not only interfere with the production of the
body's own estrogen, but also cause functional hypothyroidism
at the cellular level, due to the receptor-blocking capabilities.

There are concerns for adult consumption of soy products.
One UK study gave premenopausal women 60 grams of soy
protein per day for one month. The soy was found to disrupt
the menstrual cycle, with the effects of the isoflavones continuing for a full three months after it was removed from the
diet. Another study found that intake of soy over a long period
causes enlargement of the thyroid and suppresses thyroid function. Another study found that high soy intake in premenopausal women could suppress ovarian production of the key
reproductive hormones estradiol and progesterone by as much
as 20 to 50 percent in some women. Overconsumption of isoflavones is also thought to negatively affect fertility, and can
have serious health effects—including infertility, thyroid disease, or liver disease—in a number of mammals.

In a letter to the Food and Drug Administration dated
February 18, 1999, Doerge and Daniel Sheehan, FDA experts
on soy at the time, protested the FDA's health claims for soy
products.

There is abundant evidence that some of the isoflavones found in soy, including genistein and equol, a metabolize of daidzen, demonstrate toxicity in estrogen sensitive tissues and in the thyroid. This is true for a number of species, including humans. Additionally, isoflavones are inhibitors of the thyroid peroxidase, which makes T3 and T4. Inhibition can be expected to generate thyroid abnormalities, including goiter and autoimmune thyroiditis. There exists a significant body of animal data that demonstrates goitrogenic and even carcinogenic effects of soy products. Moreover, there are significant reports of goitrogenic effects from soy consumption in human infants and adults.

Naturopathic doctor and hormone educator Sherrill Sellman is also concerned about the use of soy.

It is now known that soy, in its unfermented forms, does have an inhibiting effect on the thyroid. Contrary to the popular myth, Asians do not eat soy as a staple food but rather only as a condiment. I have found soy to generally be a very allergic food, and unless it's fermented, it's difficult to digest. I discourage use of soy, unless it's fermented, and I'm definitely not a fan of the soy pills, soy powders, and soy protein bars.

If you want to eat soy, then tempeh, soy sauce, and miso are far more easily digested and less likely to cause problems. Soy pills, powders, and especially high-isoflavone supplements, as well as daily overconsumption of high levels of soy foods, all may contribute to the worsening of your thyroid problem and imbalance in your hormone levels.

Blair shares her cautionary tale. She had gotten her thyroid under control and lost 40 pounds, when she decided to try soy.

I started reading about soy for perimenopausal women. I actually didn't like soy. Tofu was interesting if it was fried with some sauces, but the idea of soy always seemed strange to me. I like real food and I am a good cook. What fascinated me about the soy is that it has a very high protein content and was the only bean with a complex of amino acids that were similar to those found in meat, eggs and dairy. *The Zone* diet calls for high amounts of protein throughout the day if you're exercising. I started to incorporate soy into my diet a little at a time, getting used to the tastes and textures. I found lots of recipes and began to create a new diet. My new doctor, who was an osteopath and did craniosacral manipulation, saw me starting a few months before soy and for the next three years. I started out healthier with high intent to achieve total weight loss: I had lost 40 pounds, now let's go for the next 30. She encouraged me to search the Internet and of course, all the soy articles, both scientific and lay, were selling soy as the new manna from the gods. Given my awful menstrual cycles, I'd try anything.

The weight loss soon stopped and I plateaued for three long miserable years. In the town where I lived, we loved to go up and down the hills of the river valley. These treks got harder and I noticed my legs aching for hours after. Sometimes I cried trying to make it uphill, that's how dedicated I was to my exercise routine. Autumn and winter came, I couldn't maintain my body temperature and had difficulty exercising outdoors. I would shiver so violently that I'd jump in the shower to warm up. I kept a wool blanket in the car all seasons. I had so much pain in my body that getting a good night's sleep became impossible. I noticed that while I could endure the aches and pains, what was most disturbing was my emotional state. I knew that perimenopause was an emotional time but this was way beyond what I had ever experienced. I thought I was dying. My periods became worse, closer together and more painful. I found it difficult to talk and express myself. I had pain and numbness in my arms and feet, difficulty walking at times, stumbling, even drooling! I thought I was losing my mind with the mental confusion and apathy.

Then I found Mary Shomon's article on the dangers of soy for thyroid patients. I was absolutely shocked. What had I done to myself? As I read the article and read the list of hypothyroid symptoms, I was aghast! My doctors had kept *all* this information from me *all* these years, and wasn't I a dummy for believing the media hype! I threw all the soy milk, soy burgers, soy cheese, soy powder, protein bars, soy in cereal, soy nuts and tempeh into the trash. I kept the soy sauce, because I read that the fermentation was the key to blocking the goitrogens. What a waste of money expensive soy products were. What a waste of three years of my life to be so manipulated by the soy industry.

I had regularly scheduled blood tests about a month after I quit the soy. I told my osteopath what I had learned and she was shocked, too, because she could see I was already feeling amazingly better. When the blood tests came back, my TSH had dropped from the top of the range to the bottom. I felt like a rejuvenated woman and ready to get back to the land of the living. I found the thyroid forum soon after and vowed to tell my story as often as necessary. Too many women and men are being duped by the soy industry to believe that animal fodder is human fodder.

## Chapter 5

# Thyroid Risks and Symptoms Checklist

> Knowledge comes by eyes always open and working hands; and
> there is no knowledge that is not power.
>
> —Ralph Waldo Emerson

There are a number of factors that can increase your risk of having a thyroid condition. There are also a number of factors that may trigger thyroid problems or make you more susceptible to developing a thyroid condition. I've summarized those risk factors and triggers here in this checklist, together with the symptoms that are associated with thyroid conditions. I suggest you make a copy of this checklist and fill it out. Then, you can bring it to your physician to help in getting an initial evaluation and diagnosis. If you have already been diagnosed with thyroid disease but continue to have symptoms, use the checklist to discuss the need for changes to your treatment.

For a more in-depth discussion of the particular risks and symptoms of hypothyroidism, hyperthyroidism, and autoimmune diseases, you may want to check out my other books, *Living Well with Hypothyroidism*, *Living Well with Graves' Disease and Hyperthyroidism*, and *Living Well with Autoimmune Disease*.

## Risk Factors for Thyroid Disease

### Gender
____ Female: Women are at greater risk than men.

### Age
____ I am over 50. Women 50 and above are at the highest risk, though thyroid disease can strike at any age.

### Thyroid History
____ A doctor has prescribed thyroid hormone for me in the past.
____ I have a female relative (mother, grandmother, sister, daughter) with a past or current thyroid condition.
____ I have a female relative who has tested positive for thyroid antibodies.
____ My family and I have the following thyroid history:

| | Myself | First-Degree Relative (parent, sibling, child) |
| --- | --- | --- |
| Goiter and/or benign thyroid nodules | _____ | _____ |
| Graves' disease or hyperthyroidism | _____ | _____ |
| Hashimoto's disease or hypothyroidism | _____ | _____ |
| Partial or full thyroidectomy | _____ | _____ |
| Postpartum thyroiditis | _____ | _____ |
| Radioactive iodine (RAI) treatment | _____ | _____ |
| Tested positive for thyroid antibodies | _____ | _____ |

Thyroid cancer             _____  _____
Transient thyroiditis      _____  _____

## Thyroid Hormone Exposure

\_\_\_ I recently refilled my thyroid hormone medication prescription, had it filled at a different pharmacy, or changed thyroid medication brands.

\_\_\_ I am taking more thyroid hormone medication than has been prescribed.

\_\_\_ I am taking thyroid hormone medication that has not been prescribed to me by a doctor.

\_\_\_ I take over-the-counter thyroid support supplements or thyroid glandular supplements.

\_\_\_ I take over-the-counter diet supplements.

\_\_\_ I take over-the-counter energy supplements.

\_\_\_ I regularly eat meat that has been privately butchered or is from small farms.

\_\_\_ I regularly eat game meat from hunting.

## Polyglandular Autoimmune Syndromes

\_\_\_ My family and/or I have one or more of the conditions associated with type 1 polyglandular autoimmune syndrome.

|  | Myself | First-Degree Relative (parent, sibling, child) |
|---|---|---|
| Addison's disease | _____ | _____ |
| Alopecia (hair loss) | _____ | _____ |
| Candidiasis | _____ | _____ |
| Chronic active hepatitis | _____ | _____ |
| Hyperthyroidism, thyroiditis, hypothyroidism | _____ | _____ |

Malabsorption syndrome _____ _____
Parathyroid gland failure _____ _____
Pernicious anemia _____ _____
Pituitary gland failure _____ _____
Premature menopause _____ _____
Type 1 diabetes _____ _____
Vitiligo _____ _____

——— My family and/or I have one or more of the condition associated with type 2 polyglandular autoimmune syndrome.

|  | Myself | First-Degree Relative (parent, sibling, child) |
|---|---|---|
| Addison's disease | _____ | _____ |
| Alopecia | _____ | _____ |
| Celiac disease | _____ | _____ |
| Hyperthyroidism, thyroiditis, hypothyroidism | _____ | _____ |
| Myasthenia gravis | _____ | _____ |
| Parathyroid gland failure | _____ | _____ |
| Parkinson's disease | _____ | _____ |
| Pernicious anemia | _____ | _____ |
| Premature menopause | _____ | _____ |
| Type 1 diabetes | _____ | _____ |
| Vitiligo | _____ | _____ |

### Autoimmune or Endocrine Risk Factors and History

____ I am left-handed or ambidextrous (factors associated with a higher level of autoimmune disorders than the general population).

____ I am prematurely gray-haired (factor more common in people who have an autoimmune condition versus the general population)

____ There is a history of autoimmune or endocrine disease in my family, as follows.

|  | Myself | First-Degree Relative (parent, sibling, child) |
|---|---|---|
| Adrenal problems (Addison's, Cushing's, or Turner syndrome; adrenal insufficiency; pheochromocytoma; other adrenal problems) | _____ | _____ |
| Alopecia | _____ | _____ |
| Autoimmune hypoparathyroidism | _____ | _____ |
| Autoimmune oophoritis | _____ | _____ |
| Celiac disease or gluten intolerance | _____ | _____ |
| Chronic fatigue syndrome (CFS/CFIDS) | _____ | _____ |
| Fibromyalgia | _____ | _____ |
| Growth hormone imbalances (dwarfism, deficiency, others) | _____ | _____ |
| Guillain-Barré syndrome | _____ | _____ |
| Inflammatory bowel disease | _____ | _____ |
| Juvenile rheumatoid arthritis | _____ | _____ |
| Ménière's disease | _____ | _____ |
| Multiple sclerosis | _____ | _____ |
| Osteoporosis | _____ | _____ |
| Pancreatic problems (hypoglycemia, insulin resistance, metabolic syndrome) | _____ | _____ |

Parathyroid conditions
(hyperparathyroidism, others)     _____    _____

Pernicious anemia     _____    _____

Pituitary diseases (acromegaly,
prolactinoma, pituitary
tumor, others)     _____    _____

Polycystic ovary syndrome     _____    _____

Premature ovarian decline
or failure     _____    _____

Psoriasis     _____    _____

Raynaud's syndrome     _____    _____

Rheumatoid arthritis     _____    _____

Sarcoidosis     _____    _____

Scleroderma     _____    _____

Sex hormone imbalances
(polycystic ovary syndrome,
premature menopause,
infertility, menstrual disorders)     _____    _____

Sjögren's syndrome     _____    _____

Systemic lupus erythematosus
(SLE)     _____    _____

Type 1 diabetes     _____    _____

Vitiligo     _____    _____


## Trigger Conditions

I have been diagnosed with:

\_\_\_ Celiac disease or gluten intolerance

\_\_\_ Choriocarcinoma

\_\_\_ Molar pregnancy

\_\_\_ Pituitary adenoma

\_\_\_ Struma ovarii

## Related Conditions

I have the following conditions (sometimes associated with thyroid disease):

\_\_\_ Alopecia

\_\_\_ Anemia

\_\_\_ Attention deficit hyperactivity disorder (ADHD)

\_\_\_ Bipolar disease

\_\_\_ Bipolar disorder or manic depression

\_\_\_ Candidiasis, yeast overgrowth

\_\_\_ Carpal tunnel syndrome or tendonitis

\_\_\_ Chronic Epstein-Barr virus (EBV)

\_\_\_ Chronic fatigue syndrome

\_\_\_ Chronic headaches, migraine disease

\_\_\_ Chronic premenstrual syndrome (PMS)

\_\_\_ Clinical depression

\_\_\_ Depression

\_\_\_ Down syndrome

\_\_\_ Eczema

\_\_\_ Endometriosis

\_\_\_ Generalized anxiety disorder

\_\_\_ Fibromyalgia

\_\_\_ Gynecomastia

\_\_\_ Hemochromatosis

\_\_\_ Hidradinitis suppurativa (painful, inflamed armpit and groin boils)

\_\_\_ Infertility

\_\_\_ Insulin resistance

\_\_\_ Metabolic syndrome

\_\_\_ Mitral valve prolapse (heart murmur, palpitations)

\_\_\_ Mononucleosis

\_\_\_ Ovarian cysts

\_\_\_ Panic attacks

____ Panic disorder

____ Phobias

____ Plantar's fasciitis

____ Polycystic ovary syndrome

____ Psoriasis

____ Recurrent miscarriage

____ Sleep apnea and/or snoring

____ Tarsal tunnel syndrome

____ Type 1 diabetes

____ Type 2 diabetes

____ Urticaria (hives)

____ Vitiligo

## Infection

____ I have recently had the following viral infections:

Adenovirus                          ____

Cat scratch fever                   ____

Cold                                ____

Coxsackie virus                     ____

Influenza                           ____

Measles                             ____

Mononucleosis                       ____

Mumps                               ____

Myocarditis                         ____

Upper respiratory infection         ____

____ I have recently been diagnosed with *Yersinia enterocolitica* (food-based infection).

____ I have recently eaten raw or undercooked poultry.

____ I have recently drunk unpasteurized milk and/or dairy products.

____ I have recently eaten seafood, particularly oysters, from potentially contaminated waters.

____ I have frequent infections, or infections that last a long time.

____ I get recurrent sinus infections.

### Fertility

____ I have a history of infertility.

____ I have had more than one miscarriage.

### Pregnancy History

____ I had a baby in the last 12 months.

____ I have just had a miscarriage or terminated a pregnancy.

____ I am currently pregnant.

____ I have recently been diagnosed with a molar pregnancy.

____ I have recently been diagnosed with choriocarcinoma.

____ I have delivered a stillborn baby in the past.

____ I have delivered a baby prematurely in the past.

### Menstrual Periods

____ My periods are irregular.

____ I have a very short (18 days) or very long (40 days) cycle.

____ I have very heavy or very light menstrual periods.

### Smoking

____ I've recently quit smoking.

____ I am currently a smoker.

____ I smoked in the distant past.

### Exposure to or Imbalances in Iodine

____ I recently had an X-ray or scan that used iodine contrast dye.

____ I recently had a medical procedure involving a topical antiseptic (povidone or iodine).

____ I take the heart drug Amiodarone.

____ I take iodine supplements, in pill or liquid form.

____ I take the following supplements, or combination supplements that include as an ingredient:

    Bladderwrack (fucus vesiculosus)    ____

    Bugleweed    ____

    Irish moss    ____

    Kelp    ____

    Kelp fronds    ____

    Norwegian kelp    ____

    Seaweed    ____

____ I have used Cellasene or other iodine-rich cellulite remedies.

____ I eat large amounts of seaweed.

____ I have eliminated iodized salt from my diet.

____ I live in the "goiter belt" (mountainous or inland areas,
including the Alps, Pyrenees, Himalayas, Andes,
St. Lawrence River valley, Appalachian Mountains,
Great Lakes basin westward through Minnesota, South
and North Dakota, Montana, Wyoming, southern
Canada, the Rockies, and into noncoastal Oregon,
Washington, and British Columbia).

____ My mother was iodine-deficient, had a goiter, or lived in
a goiter belt area when pregnant with me.

## Medical/Drug Treatments

____ I have recently had a medical test that involved an iodine
contrast dye.

____ I am currently or have recently been treated with inter-
feron beta-1b.

____ I am currently or have recently been treated with inter-
leukin-4.

____ I am currently or have recently been treated with immu-
nosuppressant therapy.

\_\_\_\_ I am currently being treated with antiretroviral treatment for AIDS.

\_\_\_\_ I am currently or have recently been treated with monoclonal antibody (Campath-1h) therapy for multiple sclerosis.

\_\_\_\_ I have recently received a donated organ.

\_\_\_\_ I have recently received a bone marrow transplant.

\_\_\_\_ In the past, I have taken the following drugs:

    Lithium     \_\_\_\_

    Amiodarone (Cordarone), for arrhythmia     \_\_\_\_

I am currently taking the following drugs:

    Aminoglutethimide, for breast and
    prostate cancer treatment     \_\_\_\_

    Amiodarone (Cordarone), for arrhythmia     \_\_\_\_

    Amphetamines     \_\_\_\_

    Birth control pills     \_\_\_\_

    Carbamazepine, oxcarbazepine,
    and valproate, for epilepsy     \_\_\_\_

    Cimetidine or ranitidine (Tagamet or Zantac)
    for ulcer treatment     \_\_\_\_

    Clomiphene (Clomid), for fertility treatments \_\_\_\_

    Estrace, Estraderm, Estratest, Premarin, Cenestin
    (estrogen hormone replacement products)     \_\_\_\_

    Glucocorticoids or adrenal steroids like
    prednisone and hydrocortisone     \_\_\_\_

    Ketoconazole, an antifungal     \_\_\_\_

    L-dopa inhibitors such as chlorpromazine
    (Thorazine) or haloperidol (Haldol), for psychotic
    disorders     \_\_\_\_

    Lithium     \_\_\_\_

    Metoclopramide (Reglan) and domperidone,
    for nausea or vomiting     \_\_\_\_

Para-aminosalicylic acid, a tuberculosis drug  ___
Propranolol, a beta blocker, for high blood
pressure or heart rhythm abnormalities      ___
Raloxifene (Evista), for osteoporosis        ___
Sulfonamide drugs, including sulfadiazine,
sulfasoxazole, and acetazoleamide, used as
diuretics and antibiotics                    ___
Sulfonylureas, including tolbutamide and
chlorpropamide, for diabetes                 ___

## Diet

___ I regularly consume substantial quantities of the following "goitrogenic" foods in a raw form: African cassava,
babassu, broccoli, brussels sprouts, cabbage, carrots, corn,
cauliflower, horseradish, kale, kohlrabi, millet, mustard,
mustard greens, peaches, peanuts, radishes, soy products,
spinach, strawberries, turnips, walnuts, watercress.

___ I regularly use aspartame (Nutrasweet).

___ I regularly eat foods or drink diet drinks that contain
aspartame.

___ I frequently eat fish that contain higher levels of mercury,
including:

Mackerel      ___
Shark         ___
Swordfish     ___
Tuna          ___

## Soy Overexposure

___ I was given soy formula heavily or exclusively as an infant.

___ I eat substantial quantities of soy foods: tofu, tempeh,
soy milk, soy nuts, edamame on a daily or almost daily
basis.

\_\_\_ I regularly use soy supplements in pill form.

\_\_\_ I regularly consume soy powders and smoothies.

\_\_\_ I use soy-based hormonal creams.

## Snakebite

\_\_\_ I have had a severe or life-threatening snakebite in the past. (In rare circumstances, severe snakebite can negatively affect the hypothalamus and trigger thyroid problems.)

## Trauma

\_\_\_ I have recently had my thyroid or neck area vigorously manipulated or palpated.

\_\_\_ I have recently had surgery on the thyroid, parathyroids, or the area surrounding the thyroid.

\_\_\_ I recently had a biopsy of the thyroid.

\_\_\_ I recently had an injection to the thyroid (percutaneous ethanol injection [PEI]).

\_\_\_ I recently injured my neck (whiplash, broken neck, car accident).

\_\_\_ I was recently injured by an automobile seat belt after a crash.

## Allergies and Sensitivities

\_\_\_ I have seasonal allergies, especially to pollen and trees.

\_\_\_ I have food allergies.

\_\_\_ I have been diagnosed with gluten intolerance or celiac disease.

\_\_\_ My allergies have become worse recently.

## Toxic or Environmental Exposures

\_\_\_ I have mercury dental fillings.

\_\_\_ I am exposed—through work or other means—to higher-than-usual levels of gold, cadmium, and other heavy metals.

\_\_\_ I live near a plant that produces rockets or rocket fuel, or my work exposes me to the chemical perchlorate.

\_\_\_ I drink water that comes from the Colorado River.

\_\_\_ I eat produce that is irrigated with water from the Colorado River.

\_\_\_ I grew up drink fluoridated water.

\_\_\_ I use fluoridated toothpaste, and/or a fluoride mouthwash.

\_\_\_ I get fluoride treatments at the dentist.

\_\_\_ I am regularly exposed to chlorine (e.g., swim or work at a swimming pool).

\_\_\_ I live in an area that has been recently sprayed for West Nile virus.

\_\_\_ I am exposed to insecticides and pesticides.

Radiation Exposure

\_\_\_ I have been treated for Hodgkin's disease.

\_\_\_ I lived or was visiting an area affected by the Chernobyl nuclear plant accident on or in the weeks after April 26, 1986. (Areas directly affected included Belarus, Russian Federation, and Ukraine; smaller exposure was experienced by Austria, Denmark, Finland, Germany, Greece, Italy, and Poland.)

\_\_\_ I worked at or lived in the area downwind from the former nuclear weapons plant at Hanford in south-central Washington State from the 1940s to the 1960s, particularly 1955 to 1965.

\_\_\_ I live near or work at a nuclear plant or facility.

\_\_\_ I lived near or in the general region of the Nevada nuclear test site in the 1950s and 1960s.(According to the National Cancer Institute, the highest per capita

THYROID RISKS AND SYMPTOMS CHECKLIST

thyroid doses of radiation were experienced in Utah, Idaho, Montana, Colorado, and Missouri.)

\_\_\_ I have had radiation or X-ray treatments to treat tonsils, adenoids, lymph nodes, thymus gland, Hodgkin's disease, or acne.

\_\_\_ I have had radiation treatment to my head, neck, or chest.

\_\_\_ I have had numerous X-ray treatments (not including dental or diagnostic X-rays) to the head and neck.

\_\_\_ I had nasal radium therapy sometime during the 1940s and the 1960s, as a treatment for tonsillitis, colds, or pressure changes.

## Stress

In the last year, I have experienced one or more of the following high-stress events in my life:

\_\_\_ Death of spouse

\_\_\_ Divorce

\_\_\_ Marital separation

\_\_\_ Jail term

\_\_\_ Death of close family member

\_\_\_ Personal injury or illness

\_\_\_ Marriage

\_\_\_ Fired from work

\_\_\_ Marital reconciliation

\_\_\_ Retirement

\_\_\_ Change in family member's health

\_\_\_ Pregnancy

\_\_\_ Sex difficulties

\_\_\_ Addition to family

\_\_\_ Business readjustment

\_\_\_ Change in financial status

____ Death of a close friend
____ Change in number of marital arguments
____ Mortgage or loan greater than $10,000
____ Foreclosure of mortgage or loan

## Symptoms of Thyroid Disease

### Thyroid, Throat, Neck, Mouth

____ I have a goiter.
____ My thyroid or neck is enlarged.
____ I can feel a lump—or what appears to be some sort of fullness or growth—in my neck or thyroid area.
____ I have enlarged and/or tender lymph nodes.
____ I find neckties, turtlenecks, necklaces, or neck scarves uncomfortable.
____ I have a feeling of neck or throat pressure or fullness.
____ I have a strange "buzzy" feeling in my neck or thyroid area.
____ I sometimes feel like I am choking or have something stuck in my throat.
____ Sometimes it's hard to swallow.
____ My tongue feels thick and/or trembles.
____ I have pain and tenderness in my neck and/or thyroid area.
____ My voice has become hoarse, husky, or gravelly.

### Weight and Appetite Changes

____ I feel thirsty much of the time.
____ I am unusually hungry.
____ I have no appetite.
____ I am losing weight, even though I haven't changed my diet and exercise.
____ I have experienced rapid and/or dramatic weight loss without particularly dieting.

\_\_\_ I am able to eat substantially more and not gain weight.

\_\_\_ I am able to eat more and am still losing weight.

\_\_\_ I can't gain weight, even if I eat more.

\_\_\_ I am gaining weight without a change in diet or exercise.

\_\_\_ I am unable to lose weight, despite proper diet and exercise.

\_\_\_ I am losing weight during pregnancy.

\_\_\_ I am having excessive vomiting and nausea—accompanied by weight loss—in pregnancy.

\_\_\_ I have had a baby in the last year and experienced a rapid and/or dramatic weight loss without dieting.

\_\_\_ I have recently been diagnosed as anorexic.

\_\_\_ I am craving and/or eating more carbohydrates (bread, rice, pasta, sweets, fruits, sugary foods, etc.).

\_\_\_ I'm a diabetic, and having symptoms of poor blood sugar control (hunger, shakiness when hungry).

## Ascites or Fluid in the Abdomen

\_\_\_ I have rapidly gained weight in the abdominal area.

\_\_\_ I am experiencing abdominal discomfort and distention.

\_\_\_ I'm experiencing shortness of breath.

\_\_\_ My ankles are swollen.

## Temperature

\_\_\_ I am very intolerant of any temperature extremes—hot or cold.

\_\_\_ I have a low-grade fever.

\_\_\_ I have been diagnosed as having hypothermia (low body temperature).

\_\_\_ I feel cold, especially in the hands and/or feet.

\_\_\_ My normal basal body temperature is below 97.8 degrees Fahrenheit.

____ I feel warm or hot when others are cold, or cold when others are warm.

____ I'm experiencing hot flashes.

____ I sweat excessively, or much less than normal.

____ I'm frequently thirsty.

## Heart

____ My pulse rate is particularly low or high (____ beats per minute).

____ I have unusually low or high blood pressure.

____ I feel like my heart is racing or pounding.

____ I feel like I can "hear" my heartbeat in my head.

____ I feel heart palpitations, flutters, skipped beats, strange patterns or rhythms.

____ I have frequent headaches.

____ I often feel breathless.

____ I frequently feel dizzy.

____ I have occasional chest pain.

## Gastrointestinal System

____ I have more frequent bowel movements.

____ My bowel movements are looser than normal.

____ I have diarrhea.

____ I have constipation.

____ I have to urinate more frequently.

____ I am experiencing nausea and/or vomiting.

____ I have pain in the upper right abdominal area.

## Breathing

____ I experience periods of shortness of breath.

____ I have tightness in the chest.

____ Occasionally, I feel the need to yawn to get oxygen.

Dizziness

____ I have vertigo and dizziness.

____ I sometimes feel light-headed.

Energy, Muscles, Joints

____ I feel fatigued more than normal.

____ I feel weak, run down, sluggish, lethargic.

____ I feel like I can't get enough sleep.

____ My muscles feel weak.

____ My arms, shoulders, and/or legs feel weak.

____ I have experienced one or more episodes of extreme weakness or difficulty walking.

____ I have had an unusual increase in energy.

____ I'm feeling a need to exercise far more than usual.

____ I need very little sleep.

____ I have pains, aches, and stiffness in various joints, hands, and feet.

____ I am more fatigued and sore than normal after exercise.

____ I have developed carpal tunnel syndrome, (can affect hands or forearms); my existing condition is getting worse.

____ I have developed tarsal tunnel syndrome (legs); my existing condition is getting worse.

____ I have developed plantar's fasciitis (balls of feet); my existing condition is getting worse.

Slowness

____ My movements are slower than normal.

____ My speech is slower than normal.

Skin and Face

____ My skin is smoother, younger-looking, and/or velvety.

____ I have worsening acne, breakouts.

____ My mucous membranes (mouth, eyes) are especially dry.

____ I have a dull facial expression.

____ I have puffiness around my eyes and face.

____ My skin is rough, coarse, dry, scaly, itchy, and thick.

____ I get painful, inflamed boils in my armpits or groin.

____ I'm bruising easily.

____ I have prominent spider veins on my face and neck.

____ I have blister-like bumps on my forehead and face.

____ My face, throat, palms, and elbows have a flushed appearance.

____ My coloring is pale; my lips are pale.

____ My skin is yellowish.

____ I get hives frequently.

____ I experience itching.

____ I have patches of unpigmented skin (vitiligo).

____ I have waxy, reddish-brown lesions on my lower legs, feet, toes, arms, face, shoulders, or trunk.

____ I have swollen eyelids.

## Hair Changes

____ My hair is falling out more than usual.

____ I'm losing body hair.

____ I'm losing hair from the outer edge of my eyebrows.

____ My hair has become thinner.

____ My hair has become finer.

____ My hair has become softer.

____ My hair can no longer hold a perm or a curl.

____ My hair has become rough and coarse.

____ My hair has become dry.

____ My hair has been breaking and has become brittle.

## Nails and Hands

____ My nails are more shiny than usual.

____ My nails are dry and more brittle and break more easily.

____ My nails are softer.

____ My hands and palms are warm and moist.

____ My nail bed is separating from my finger.

____ I have swollen hands.

____ I have pain in the joints of my fingers.

### Legs, Feet, Toes

____ My toes are swelling and becoming wider.

____ I have pain in the joints of my toes.

____ I have swollen feet.

____ I have tarsal tunnel syndrome (pain in leg).

____ I have plantar's fasciitis (pain in the balls of the feet).

____ I have waxy, reddish-brown lesions on my lower legs, feet, toes.

### Eyes

____ My eyes feel uncomfortable.

____ My eyes feel dry, and gritty.

____ It feels as if there is something in my eye.

____ My eyes are tearing and watering frequently.

____ There are visible blood vessels in my eyes.

____ My upper and lower eyelids look irritated and puffy.

____ I feel an achiness or pain behind my eyes.

____ I frequently have a headache in the eye area.

____ My eyeballs are bulging or protruding.

____ I can't completely close my eye during sleep.

____ I have a noticeable "stare."

____ My upper eyelids are retracting, giving me a wide-eyed, startled look.

____ I have tics, twitches, and tremors in my eyes or eyelids.

____ I don't blink frequently.

____ My eyes get jumpy (tics in eyes).

\_\_\_\_ When I shift my gaze quickly, I feel dizzy or disoriented.

\_\_\_\_ My vision is blurred or worsening.

\_\_\_\_ My vision is blurry, but eyedrops help.

\_\_\_\_ I find colors are less vivid and brightness is diminishing.

\_\_\_\_ I have double vision.

\_\_\_\_ I have poor night vision.

\_\_\_\_ I'm light-sensitive.

\_\_\_\_ I see "flashing lights" or floaters.

\_\_\_\_ My eyelids are puffy.

### Hearing/Tinnitus

\_\_\_\_ I have tinnitus (ringing in ears).

\_\_\_\_ I have sudden hearing loss or onset of deafness.

### Mood, Thinking, Cognition

\_\_\_\_ My moods change easily.

\_\_\_\_ My mind feels like I'm in a fog.

\_\_\_\_ I find it difficult to focus or concentrate.

\_\_\_\_ I find it difficult to make decisions.

\_\_\_\_ I'm feeling confused and my thinking is disorganized.

\_\_\_\_ I have dyslexia.

\_\_\_\_ I'm having difficulty with reading or calculating.

\_\_\_\_ I have memory problems, and am forgetting things more frequently.

\_\_\_\_ I feel like my mind is going blank regularly.

\_\_\_\_ My mind is always racing; I can't shut my thoughts off.

### Depression

\_\_\_\_ I feel sad, empty, worthless, or hopeless.

\_\_\_\_ I feel hopeless or pessimistic.

\_\_\_\_ I feel guilty or helpless.

\_\_\_\_ I am withdrawing emotionally.

____ I've lost interest or pleasure in activities and hobbies.

____ I've lost interest or pleasure in sex.

____ I have thoughts of death or suicide.

____ I have mood swings.

____ I'm feeling unusually elated.

____ I'm feeling unusually self-confident.

____ I'm having hallucinations.

____ I'm taking an antidepressant, but it doesn't seem to be working.

## Anxiety and Panic

____ I feel that sometimes I am behaving erratically or over-emotionally.

____ I feel uncontrollable and/or irrational anger or aggressiveness at times when it's not appropriate.

____ I feel anxious, nervous, restless, irritable, and on edge.

____ I feel inexplicably frightened at times.

____ I find it hard to stop worrying.

____ I'm jumpy, easily startled.

____ My reflexes are particularly fast.

____ I have tremors.

____ My hands are shaky.

____ I'm always moving, jiggling, tapping a foot, drumming my fingers—can't sit still.

____ I have panic attacks.

## Sleep Problems

____ I find it hard to fall asleep.

____ After I've fallen asleep, I frequently wake up.

____ When I wake up in the middle of the night, I find it hard to fall back asleep.

____ I have insomnia and can't sleep.

____ I wake feeling tired and unrefreshed.

____ I frequently oversleep.

____ I am frequently exhausted.

____ I snore.

____ I have sleep apnea.

## Menstruation

____ My premenstrual symptoms seems to have gotten worse.

____ My menstrual periods have stopped.

____ My menstrual periods have become unusually light.

____ My menstrual periods have become unusually short.

____ My menstrual periods are coming less frequently.

____ My menstrual periods have become unusually heavy.

____ My menstrual periods have become unusually long.

____ My menstrual periods are coming more frequently.

## Sex Drive

____ My sex drive is low or nonexistent.

____ I have difficulty reaching orgasm.

____ I suddenly have a "raging libido" or unusually high sex drive.

____ I'm behaving in a sexually obsessive way.

____ I have constant excessive vaginal lubrication.

## Fertility

____ I'm unable to get pregnant.

____ I've had a miscarriage or multiple miscarriages.

____ I'm showing signs that I'm not ovulating.

____ I have an in vitro fertilization failure.

____ I've had donor egg failure.

## Symptoms in Pregnancy

____ I am vomiting excessively.

\_\_\_ I am losing weight or not gaining appropriately.

\_\_\_ I have an extreme case of morning sickness.

\_\_\_ I am gaining excessive weight during pregnancy.

\_\_\_ I am extremely fatigued.

\_\_\_ My hair is falling out.

\_\_\_ I'm feeling unusually depressed.

## Postpartum Symptoms

\_\_\_ I have had or am having difficulty breastfeeding.

\_\_\_ I am having difficulty losing weight.

\_\_\_ I am losing large amounts of hair.

\_\_\_ I am abnormally fatigued.

\_\_\_ I'm experiencing depression and mood swings.

\_\_\_ I'm having brain fog and difficulty concentrating.

## Breast Changes

\_\_\_ My breasts are leaking milk, but I'm not lactating or breastfeeding.

## Menopause and Perimenopause

\_\_\_ My perimenopause symptoms seem to have gotten worse.

\_\_\_ My menopause symptoms seem to have gotten worse.

# Special Symptoms in Children, Preteens, and Teenagers

\_\_\_ Growth: recent sudden growth spurt, or failure to keep up with growth charts for height

\_\_\_ Early appearance of breast buds

\_\_\_ Early breast development

\_\_\_ Unusual vaginal bleeding before the first menstrual period

____ Breast discharge

____ Long gaps between menstrual periods

____ Failed to get menstrual period or secondary sexual development (breasts, underarm and pubic hair)

____ Recently developed poor handwriting

____ Poor school performance, difficulty concentrating at school

____ Diagnosis of attention deficit disorder

____ Weakness or aches in legs or arms

____ Unusual fatigue, sleeping far more than usual

____ Concern that the child may be taking illegal drugs

____ More emotional outbursts, temper tantrums

____ Onset of bedwetting

____ Can't sit still, hyperactive-like movements, including leg swinging, finger tapping, etc.

____ Concern that the child or teen may be anorexic; diagnosis of anorexia

## Special Symptoms in the Elderly/Seniors

____ Dementia, confusion, forgetfulness

____ Withdrawn, lacking in energy

____ More frequent falls and injuries

____ More shaking

# Part II

## THYROID-RELATED HORMONE ISSUES

# Chapter 6

# Puberty, Menstrual, and Sexual Problems

*Women complain about premenstrual syndrome, but I think of it as the only time of the month I can be myself.*

—Roseanne Barr

Menstrual irregularities and puberty problems frequently go hand in hand with thyroid conditions. Some studies have reported that anywhere from 50 to 80 percent of women with thyroid conditions have menstrual problems, at two to three times the rate of the general population.

Thyroid conditions are associated with more anovulatory cycles, hyperprolactinemia, and luteal phase defects. These problems can all cause early or late puberty and first menstrual period, worsened physical and emotional symptoms of menstruation, PMS, menstrual cycle length irregularities, and problems with the heaviness of the bleeding, all of which are described in this chapter. The thyroid is also linked to sex drive, and issues of how the thyroid impacts your libido and what can be done about it are discussed at the end of this section.

# Puberty Problems

## *Delayed Puberty*

Puberty is considered delayed in girls if it hasn't started by the age of 13 or if menstruation hasn't begun by the age of 16.

Some delay in puberty can be hereditary. If a girl's mother didn't start menstruating until she was 14, then there is a greater chance her daughter will also start menstruating late. This sort of normal, hereditary delay is called a "constitutional delay," and doesn't typically require any treatment. The child is developing normally, it's just on a somewhat later schedule.

Hypothyroidism can be a cause of delayed puberty. A young girl with Graves' disease or hyperthyroidism may also have delayed puberty. If menstruation began before the onset of a hyperthyroid condition, it's also fairly common for girls and young teenagers to stop menstruating as a symptom of the thyroid condition. Some children with hypothyroidism also have galactorrhea (leaking of milk from the breasts), along with classic hypothyroidism symptoms (see Chapter 5).

Delays in puberty also have medical causes besides thyroid disease. Illnesses that can delay puberty include diabetes, cystic fibrosis, kidney disease, pituitary conditions, asthma, and anorexia nervosa. Certain chromosomal disorders—for example, Turner's syndrome—can also cause delayed puberty by interfering with proper development of the ovaries and sex hormones.

Girls who are extremely physically active may be late developers because their level of exercise keeps them extremely lean; low body fat levels can affect hormone levels that trigger puberty. Girls' bodies require a certain amount of fat before they can go through puberty or get their periods.

If abnormally delayed puberty is suspected, a pediatric endocrinologist should be consulted. The various conditions that can delay puberty, including hypothyroidism or hyperthyroidism, should be ruled out. Note, however, that thyroid tests are not a routine requirement for a delayed-puberty medical evaluation. You may have to request thyroid testing specifically.

The physician should also evaluate the girl's level of exercise. The girl's growth will be charted, and typically, blood work is done for pituitary, chromosomal, and other conditions. An MRI scan of the brain and pituitary may be done if there's any suspicion of hypothalamic-pituitary problems. Some physicians also do an X-ray to assess bone age. This helps identify any growth abnormalities, which allows the doctor to see whether the bones are maturing normally.

In cases where delayed puberty is due to underlying thyroid disease, either optimal thyroid hormone replacement for hypothyroidism or appropriate hyperthyroidism treatment may be able to restore hormonal balance and allow for more normal reproductive development.

In other cases, treatments may include various drugs to stimulate sex hormone development or, more controversially, growth hormone.

### Precocious Puberty

An estimated 4 to 5 percent of girls have precocious puberty. Precocious puberty refers to the appearance of any of the following signs of puberty in a girl 7 or younger (6 in African American girls):

- Start of menstruation
- Breast development

- Pubic or underarm hair development
- Rapid height growth—a growth spurt
- Body odor

Ultimately, because the rapid growth causes bone to mature too quickly, girls with precocious puberty can also end up unusually short as adults.

Precocious puberty is triggered by the hypothalamus, which tells the pituitary to release hormones that stimulate the ovaries to make sex hormones. For the majority of girls, there's no underlying medical problem—they simply start puberty too early for no known reason. Some precocious puberty appears to be genetic, having a parent or sibling with early puberty puts a child at greater risk.

Sometimes, however, precocious puberty is triggered by, for example, a condition in the central nervous system or brain (such as a growth or tumor), head trauma, or a brain inflammation or infection (such as meningitis). In other cases, a problem in the ovaries or thyroid triggers the early puberty.

Because there is a complex but well-known link between increased body fat and early puberty, high body fat levels at a young age may also contribute to precocious puberty.

While precocious puberty is not a very common side effect of thyroid conditions, it has unique characteristics. Early breast development and menstruation are common, but girls usually do not develop underarm and pubic hair early. In thyroid-triggered precocious puberty, galactorrhea is sometimes seen, as are multicystic ovaries, observable on ultrasound tests.

The theory behind precocious puberty in hypothyroid girls is that the pituitary's release of TRH—which stimulates elevated TSH that causes hypothyroidism—may also be stimulating gonadotropins, the hormones that trigger the production of sex hormones, as well as prolactin, the hormone that stimulates milk production.

Evaluation of precocious puberty is usually done by a pediatric endocrinologist and involves blood and urine tests to evaluate various hormone levels. Imaging and scanning tests such as CT scans, MRIs, and ultrasound tests may be done to rule out tumors, cysts, and growths in the brain or ovaries.

Once precocious puberty is established, the pediatric endocrinologist's goal is to stop—or even reverse—the sexual development, stop accelerated growth, and slow down the rapid bone development that can actually stunt growth.

Typically, if there is a tumor, cyst, or growth causing the problem, that would be treated. If the problem is primarily hormonal, then high levels of sex hormones are usually lowered with drugs called luteinizing hormone-releasing hormone (LHRH) analogs—most commonly the drug Lupron, given by periodic injection. This synthetic hormone can block early production of the sex hormones that cause precocious puberty. Typically, these drugs halt the puberty and may even shrink the breasts somewhat. Growth also typically slows down to a more appropriate rate.

While proper thyroid diagnosis and treatment may help reverse the hormonal imbalance that sets precocious puberty in motion, restoration of the thyroid to normal levels may not stop the precocious puberty already under way, and LHRH analog treatment may still be necessary.

## Menstrual Problems

Most common in women with hypothyroidism are metrorrhagia, menorrhagia, and oligomenorrhea. The most common menstrual disorders in women with hyperthyroidism are oligo-menorrhea, amenorrhea, and hypomenorrhea. These are discussed in following sections of this chapter.

In women with hyperthyroidism, smoking particularly aggravates the menstrual problems, and some studies have found that among hyperthyroidism patients with menstrual problems, half are smokers.

Fran's period started at the age of 10 and caused her problems for decades.

> Throughout my adolescence and most of my childbearing years, my periods were very irregular. It was not unusual for my cycle to run anywhere from 35 days to 100 days. Then in 1990, at the age of 36, I had surgery for endometriosis and doctors thought that would help make my periods regular. It didn't. My hypothyroidism was diagnosed in 1992, when I was 38 years old. This was after 13 years of doctors trying to figure out why I felt so horrible. For 10 of those years, I was told it was probably multiple sclerosis, because all other tests were normal. After my diagnosis of hypo, there were many years of trying different dosages of T4, mostly Synthroid, but nothing helped me feel good for more than a few months at a time. Finally, in 2001, I asked my doctor if I could try some T3, which I had read about on your site. My goal was just to feel better and be able to think clearly again. It never entered my mind that suddenly, at the age of 47, I would start having regular monthly periods for the first time in my life. I'm certain it was due to the addition of T3.

### Premenstrual Syndrome

Premenstrual syndrome (PMS) is a group of symptoms that are related to the hormonal fluctuations occurring in your menstrual cycle. PMS symptoms typically occur in the week to 10 days prior to the onset of your period. Once your period starts, the symptoms usually go away.

It's estimated that as many as 70 percent of menstruating women have mild PMS symptoms, and as many as 18 percent have PMS symptoms severe enough to interfere with normal activities.

PMS is more common in women in their twenties and thirties and may improve during perimenopause, but some women have it consistently from the onset of menstruation until menopause.

*Note:* If you have had a hysterectomy but still have at least one ovary, you can still experience PMS.

Typical PMS symptoms include:

- Weight gain from fluid retention
- Breast swelling and tenderness
- Fluid retention, bloating, swelling of hands or feet
- Fatigue
- Insomnia, trouble sleeping, frequent waking
- Upset stomach, bloating, constipation, or diarrhea
- Headaches, migraines, sinus, ear or head fullness
- Backaches, abdominal pain, pelvic pain, cramps
- Appetite changes, food binges or food cravings (sweet foods, chocolate, salt)
- Joint or muscle pain
- Tension, irritability, mood swings, crying spells, outbursts, feeling out of control
- Anxiety, agitation, depression, social withdrawal, lack of motivation
- Trouble thinking, concentrating, or remembering
- Shortness of breath, asthma attacks
- Constipation, diarrhea, nausea

- Dizziness, blurred vision
- Racing heartbeat, palpitations, tremors, sweating
- Increase in acne, oiliness of skin, oiliness of hair
- Low sex drive

A small percentage of women have a severe, disabling form of PMS known as premenstrual dysphoric disorder (PMDD). Symptoms include severe depression, feelings of hopelessness, anxiety, extreme tension, and anger, as well as the common PMS physical symptoms, in most cycles for at least 12 months. It's estimated that 3 to 8 percent of women of childbearing age meet the criteria for PMDD diagnosis.

Experts don't know why some women get PMS and others don't. It may relate to sensitivity to the changes in hormones or subtle imbalances in the hormones. But we do know that sensitivity to shifting hormones during the menstrual cycle is to blame for symptoms.

## Dysmenorrhea

*Dysmenorrhea* is the term for painful periods. Primary dysmenorrhea has no specific physical abnormality as a cause. Secondary dysmenorrhea is painful periods that have a physical cause, such as endometriosis or fibroids. As many as 90 percent of women have cramps, particularly before they have their first child. Cramps are the main sign of dysmenorrhea and typically affect the lower abdomen or lower back.

As many as 10 percent of women have severe dysmenorrhea, and can't participate in normal activities. For women with severe dysmenorrhea, symptoms can include:

- Nausea and vomiting
- Loose stools

- Sweating
- Dizziness

Smoking and being overweight aggravate dysmenorrhea.

It's thought that dysmenorrhea is caused by prostaglandins, the chemicals that the body produces to make the uterine muscles contract and expel the endometrium during menstruation. Some research has shown that women with dysmenorrhea produce as much as 10 times the prostaglandin levels as women without pain. And most of the prostaglandins are released during the first 48 hours of menstruation, so pain typically begins several hours before the period begins and usually lasts no more than 3 days.

## Cycle Length Problems

Some change in cycles is normal as we age. There is a steady decline in menstrual cycle length as we get older. For example, while the overall median menstrual cycle length is 28 days, at age 40, the median declines to 27 days. The decline is thought to be linked in some way to the decline in the number of follicles remaining. In general, however, fewer than two or more than three menstrual periods in a 90-day interval in women ages 20 to 40 years is considered abnormal and requires evaluation. So does menstrual bleeding that lasts for more than 10 days.

## Oligomenorrhea and Polymenorrhea

*Oligomenorrhea* refers to cycles that are repeatedly longer than 35 days—or only four to nine periods per year. *Polymenorrhea* refers to repeated cycles of less than 21 days, or menstruation at two- to three-week intervals. In addition to hormonal imbalances, oligomenorrhea and polymenorrhea can be caused by pituitary changes, nutrition, stress, and various pelvic disorders and conditions.

Polymenorrhea is treated by improving general health, correcting anemia, treating pelvic causes (if any), and combined estrogen and progesterone therapy from day 5 to day 25 of the menstrual cycle. If medical treatment does not work, dilatation and curettage (D & C) may be suggested.

### Metrorrhagia

*Metrorrhagia* is the technical term for bleeding at irregular intervals, particularly between the expected menstrual periods. It can include everything from light spotting to heavy bleeding or bleeding that goes on for weeks.

Some spotting is, of course, normal when a woman has just started on birth control pills, at ovulation, or a few days before the period starts. Menopausal women on hormone replacement may also have some monthly bleeding, known as withdrawal bleeding. Other erratic bleeding should be evaluated, especially:

- Girls who are bleeding before puberty or onset of menstruation
- Menopausal or postmenopausal women who are not on hormone therapy
- Women who have had a hysterectomy

### Menorrhagia or Hypermenorrhea

*Menorrhagia* is not just a "heavy" period—it involves excessive or prolonged menstrual bleeding, or both. "Excessive" means soaking through at least a pad or tampon an hour for several consecutive hours. Sometimes the term *hypermenorrhea* is used; it refers to a more than 20 percent increase in the heaviness of the menstrual flow.

Menorrhagia is more common right after a girl starts menstruating and during perimenopause. Some estimates find that it occurs in 9 to 14 percent of all women.

Signs of menorrhagia include:

- Having to double up on your menstrual protection: a super tampon and a maxi pad, or two pads
- Heavy flow that requires that you change your tampon or pad at night
- A menstrual period that lasts longer than seven days
- Menstrual flow that includes large blood clots
- A menstrual period that is so heavy that it interferes with your lifestyle

Tiredness, fatigue, or shortness of breath can indicate anemia due to excessive menstrual blood loss.

Menorrhagia is the most common cause of anemia in premenopausal women, so symptoms of anemia should also be considered. Mild anemia can cause weakness and fatigue. More severe anemia can cause additional symptoms, including shortness of breath, elevated pulse rate, dizziness, headaches, ringing in the ears (tinnitus), irritability, and pale skin.

Causes of menorrhagia typically include hormone imbalances, although it can also be due to fibroids, polyps, lupus, pelvic inflammatory disease (PID), or some reproductive cancers or it can be related to IUD use.

Before being diagnosed with thyroid disease, Ellie had more than a decade of menstrual problems, including menorrhagia.

When I was a teenager I had unusually painful periods, but at the time, they were normal to me and it didn't occur to me that I could feel better. My mother used to joke that you could look at my absenteeism report from school and figure out my cycle. I'd be down for the count in pain—the cramps would debilitate me. The flow was something else again. By the time I was in my late twenties I was wearing two super tampons and a pad during the day, changing three to four times a day. I'd go to bed with the same and sleep on a towel because I knew I'd never last till morning. I ruined or stained countless pairs of underwear. It was a way of life and I knew no different.

## Amenorrhea

*Hypomenorrhea* refers to a more than 20 percent decrease in heaviness of flow, but what is more common is *amenorrhea*, the absence of menstrual periods. Amenorrhea is classified as primary (where periods have not started by the age of 16) or secondary (where menstrual periods have stopped for three to six months in a woman who previously had periods).

Amenorrhea can happen during puberty or later in life. It affects 2 to 5 percent of women of childbearing age. It's thought that as many as two-thirds of female atheletes have amenorrhea.

The most common cause of amenorrhea is pregnancy.

Another common cause of amenorrhea is anorexia or excessive exercise. In some women with anorexia, or who are athletes or exercise excessively, the ratio of body fat to weight drops so low that menstruation stops entirely. A study conducted at UC/San Francisco found that as many as 11 percent of women who are regular ultramarathon runners had amenorrhea, a much higher rate than in the general population. Ballet dancers, gymnasts, and ice skaters are reportedly particularly at risk, because they are combining highly athletic, rigorous physical exercise with a diet intended to keep them very thin. (This has led to the condition's nickname "ballerina amenorrhea.")

Other causes of amenorrhea include:

- Use of contraceptives
- Breastfeeding
- Certain medications, such as antidepressants, antipsychotics, chemotherapy drugs, and oral corticosteroids
- Androgen excess, or polycystic ovary disease
- Excessively low body weight, eating disorders
- Excessive exercise
- Pituitary tumor
- Uterine scarring
- Premature ovarian decline or failure
- History of chemotherapy or radiation therapy
- Adrenal insufficiency
- Sarcoidosis
- Hemachromatosis
- Stress, psychiatric disorders such as depression, obsessive-compulsive disorder, or schizophrenia
- Autoimmune endocrine disorders: hyperthyroidism, hypothyroidism, or autoimmune lymphocytic hypophysitis, Cushing syndrome, pheochromocytoma
- Drug abuse with cocaine and opioids
- Alcoholism
- AIDS, HIV disease, or other immune-deficiency conditions
- Cancer

## Medical Evaluation of Menstrual Problems

Evaluation of menstrual problems requires that your doctor take a complete medical history. This should include information about your sexual development during puberty, your methods of birth control if applicable, and your mother and grandmother's puberty, menstrual, fertility and menopausal patterns.

You should note any of the following symptoms:

- Discharge from breasts
- Hot flashes
- Facial hair
- Headaches
- Impaired vision
- Recent gynecologic procedures and events
- Changes in your weight, diet, or exercise patterns

You'll also want to provide specific information about your menstrual patterns. To help your doctor, consider filling out the menstrual chart featured in the appendix.

Blood and urine tests will be done to evaluate various hormone levels: estrogen levels, FSH, LH, and prolactin.

In addition to general hormonal imbalances, one specific condition that can result in menstrual problems is polycystic ovary syndrome (PCOS), also known as Stein-Leventhal syndrome. PCOS is a condition in which the ovaries develop cysts, hormone levels are dysfunctional, and high androgens cause abdominal obesity and weight gain, increased risk of diabetes, acne, increased facial hair, and fertility problems.

The doctor should also perform a physical examination, including a pelvic exam, to look for evidence of structural or anatomic abnormalities, inflammation, polyps, cysts, tumors, infection, or other gynecologic conditions. Typically, a Pap test, and (if premenopausal) a pregnancy test are also done. Generally, the doctor will attempt to rule out the following gynecological causes for menstrual irregularities and problems:

- Vaginal infection
- Tumors, polyps, fibroids, or cysts of the vagina, cervix, uterus, ovaries, or fallopian tubes
- Cervical disorders, cervical abrasions
- Cancer of the uterus, cervix, vagina, vulva, or bladder
- Sexually transmitted diseases such as chlamydia, gonorrhea, or genital warts
- Vaginal injury from trauma or sexual abuse
- Early pregnancy-associated bleeding
- Ectopic pregnancy (where the fertilized egg becomes implanted inside the fallopian tubes or outside the uterus)
- Adenomyosis
- Endometriosis, a condition in which the tissue that normally lines the uterus grows outside the uterus
- Pelvic inflammatory disease (PID), a sexually transmitted infection
- Tipped or retroverted uterus
- Intrauterine device (IUD) for birth control
- Scarring or adhesions from earlier surgery
- Vaginal septum
- Turner's syndrome, a birth defect related to the reproductive system

Other conditions and issues that can cause or worsen menstrual irregularities include:

- Inflammatory bowel disease (IBD)
- Pituitary growth or tumor

- Other endocrine or adrenal disease, such as Cushing's disease

The doctor should also evaluate:

- Illicit use of steroids to enhance athletic performance
- Dramatic weight change
- Use of antidepressants, which can increase prolactin
- Use drugs like Thorazine and Haldol, which can elevate prolactin
- Unusual or chronic stress

Additional tests or procedures may be done:

- CT scan, to look for cysts, fibroids, tumors, and other abnormalities
- MRI, to look for cysts, fibroids, tumors, and other abnormalities
- Laparoscopy or hysteroscopy: insertion of small camera into the abdomen or uterus, for direct assessment
- Ultrasound, to look for fibroids or other abnormalities
- Endometrial biopsy, a procedure done in a doctor's office to check the health of uterine tissue
- Dilation and curettage (D and C): scraping of the uterine lining, for evaluation

## Prescription Treatments

### Oral Contraceptives

Oral contraceptives—often referred to as "the pill"—are drugs that contain combinations of estrogen and synthetic progesterone (progestin). In addition to serving as a birth control method, oral contraceptives can help regulate ovulation, and erratic menstrual cycles, help with pain, and cut down on situations where menstrual bleeding is heavy or prolonged. Oral contraceptives actually prevent ovulation, so they minimize a great deal of the hormonal ups and downs that can trigger symptoms.

Birth control pills can have serious side effects, so these drugs are not given to anyone with a personal or family history of blood clots, cerebrovascular disease, heart disease, and breast cancer, among other conditions. Smoking while on birth control pills also seriously increases the risk. Other side effects can include bloating, weight gain, and acne.

Some experts do not recommend use of oral contraceptives, however. According to menopause educator Pat Rackowski,

> These [oral contraceptives] may work perfectly well for some women. Let me just warn, however, that "low dose" here means lower dose than they used to be. These birth control pills still contain at least four times the amount of hormones as in postmenopausal hormone replacement therapy. Also, the oral contraceptives contain synthetic hormones, which are not an exact copy of the body's own hormones. In the case of synthetic progestins, they do not have all the beneficial effects of natural progesterone on mood, energy, and fluid balance. In fact, synthetic progestins in birth control pills and in Provera, the progestin in PremPro and PremPhase, can cause worse mood swings, fluid retention, and fatigue than you had before. In both cases, I recommend natural estrogen and progesterone.

A special note for thyroid patients: If you start birth control pills, you may need an increase in your dose of thyroid hormone. Be sure to have thyroid function, including TSH and free T4, retested no later than 12 weeks after starting the contraceptive pill.

### Progestins and Progesterone

Progestins—synthetic progesterone—are sometimes prescribed as a way to bring on a woman's period. Such medications include medroxyprogesterone (Provera, Depo-Provera), norethindrone acetate (Aygestin, Norlutate), and norgestrel (Ovrel).

Natural progesterone is also available by prescription, including the manufactured product Prometrium, which is oral micronized progesterone. Compounding pharmacies can also produce compounded progesterone capsules and progesterone vaginal suppositories.

### Synthetic Gonadotropin-Releasing Hormone

In some cases, synthetic hormones such as nafarelin (Synarel) and leuprolide (Lupron) are given. These drugs are more potent versions of natural gonadotropin-releasing hormone. They can help prevent ovulation, and therefore reduce symptoms, but the patient ceases to have periods.

### Danazol

Danazol (brand name Danocrine) is a synthetic androgen, or male sex hormone, that blocks the production of certain female hormones. Danazol is sometimes helpful for severe menorrhagia, but because the drug has significant side effects, including blood clots and stroke, severe liver disease, intra-abdominal hemorrhage, and benign intracranial hypertension (pseudotumor cerebri), it is falling out of favor.

## Menotropins and Nonsteroidal Ovulatory Stimulants

Menotropins (FSH and LH) and nonsteroidal ovulatory stimulants—known as fertility drugs—can help induce ovulation, which may help regulate erratic cycles in some women.

When a woman is not ovulating regularly and trying to conceive, ovulation is induced by the nonsteroidal ovulatory stimulants called clomiphene (Clomid or Serophene). When clomiphene is ineffective, a menotropin (Menopur, Repronex, Pergonal, Humegon) is given by daily injection. Menotropins cause more than one egg to be released at a time, and can cause multiple births.

## Prescription Anti-inflammatory Drugs

COX-2 inhibitors are prescription nonsteroidal anti-inflammatory drugs (NSAIDs) that were thought to have less risk of causing stomach problems or ulcers. They have, however, been found to cause serious side effects. Two of the three popular COX-2 inhibitors—rofecoxib (Vioxx) and valdecoxib (Bextra)—have been taken off the market by the FDA, leaving only celecoxib (Celebrex). This drug is prescribed only if over-the-counter NSAIDs are not effective, and no other contraindications exist.

## Anti-anxiety Drugs

For women who suffer from irritability, anxiety, and severe mood changes, anti-anxiety drugs may be recommended. These drugs can include the benzodiazepines, which help by depressing the central nervous system. Some of the common benzodiazepines include alprazolam (Xanax), clonazepam (Klonopin), diazepam (Valium), lorazepam (Ativan), temazepam (Restoril), and triazolam (Halcion). These drugs can be addictive; they can also result in severe drowsiness in some people.

## Antidepressants

Selective serotonin reuptake inhibitors (SSRIs) can help by increasing the activity of serotonin, which may be low in women with significant menstrually related depression, anger, mood changes, and anxiety. They may also help with food cravings. In some cases, women are given the antidepressants only during the two weeks before menstruation begins.

For the more severe depression seen in PMDD, the SSRIs may be prescribed for everyday use, not just cyclically. Some women also respond to tricyclic antidepressants such as amitriptyline (Elavil, Endep), doxepin (Adapin, Sinequan), nortryptyline (Pamelor), and imipramine (Tofranil). These medicines can have significant side effects, including dizziness, drowsiness, nausea, fatigue, and weight gain. They are usually prescribed only if the SSRIs are ineffective.

## Diuretics

Diuretics, which are often referred to as "water pills," are drugs that help the body get rid of excess fluid and sodium. They can help with menstrually related weight gain, breast swelling and pain, and painful bloating. Some of the commonly prescribed diuretic drugs include spironolactone (Aldactone), triamterene (Dyazide, Maxzide), hydrochlorothiazide (Hydrodiuril) Lasix (furosemide), triamterene, and metolazone (Mykrox, Zaroxolyn).

# Medical Procedures and Surgeries

If drug therapies don't work, or the condition is due to an anatomical abnormality, tumor, or cyst, other procedures or surgery may be required.

### Removing IUD

In some cases cycle or flow irregularities or pain may be caused by an intrauterine birth control device (IUD). Removing the IUD may be recommended as part of the treatment.

### Dilation and Curettage

Dilation and curettage (D and C) involves dilating the cervix and suctioning out the uterine lining to help reduce menstrual bleeding. It does not affect the ability to become pregnant, but the procedure may have to be repeated periodically.

### Operative Hysteroscopy

Operative hysteroscopy involves use of a tiny tube known as a hysteroscope that is inserted into the uterus, to view the uterine cavity. This procedure can help visualize and surgically remove polyps that may be causing irregular or heavy menstrual bleeding.

### Endometrial Ablation

Endometrial ablation uses ultrasound to permanently destroy the endometrium—the uterine lining. After endometrial ablation, menstrual periods typically return to normal, though in a small percentage of patients, they will have little flow or complete cessation of periods. Endometrial ablation can make it difficult to become pregnant; it is usually recommended only to women who have completed their childbearing.

### Endometrial Resection

Endometrial resection involves using electrosurgical technique to remove the uterine lining. It is not typically done when a woman has fibroids, polyps, or cancer. It can help with very heavy menstrual bleeding, but as a side effect, it can affect the ability to become pregnant; therefore, endometrial resection is usually recommended only to women who have completed their childbearing.

### Hysterectomy

For irregular bleeding and periods, the most recommended procedure is hysterectomy. Hysterectomy involves surgical removal of the uterus and cervix. It's a permanent, irreversible surgery, done under general anesthesia, that causes sterility and the end of menstrual periods. An abdominal hysterectomy usually requires a five-day hospital stay; vaginal hysterectomies require stays of two to four days in the hospital.

Hysterectomy that removes the ovaries as well—known as a total hysterectomy—will usually cause premature menopause in a younger woman.

While hysterectomy may be the most recommended procedure, it's not the most preferred by patients. Various studies have shown that only 30 percent of women would want to end their periods completely through hysterectomy. Two-thirds would rather choose a treatment that would potentially reduce the bleeding without eliminating periods, including hormone treatment (62 percent), endometrial ablation (53 percent), or D and C (38 percent).

## Over-the-Counter Treatments and Supplements

Hormonal rebalancing therapy and bioidentical hormones, used to restore balance in the reproductive cycle, including the hypothalamus, pituitary, thyroid, ovarian, and adrenal glands, are described in Chapter 11.

### *Progesterone Supplements and Creams*

Over-the-counter progesterone supplements and creams are derived from wild yams and soybeans. Some physicians recommend them, and some women find them effective. There are numerous brands. One of the most recognized and reputable brands is Pro-Gest, made by Emerita.

### *PMS Drugs*

Over-the-counter PMS drugs typically combine a pain reliever with caffeine, antihistamines, or diuretics (Midol, Pamprin, and Premsyn PMS).

### *Prostaglandin Inhibitors and Nonsteroidal*
### *Anti-inflammatory Drugs*

Because so many menstrual symptoms are related to the excess of prostaglandins, drugs that inhibit prostaglandins, reduce inflammation, and help with pain may be recommended. These include nonsteroidal anti-inflammatory drugs (NSAIDs) such as ibuprofen (Advil, Motrin), and naproxen (Aleve, Naprosyn), which help reduce cramping and blood flow. Typically, these drugs should be started a day before the period is expected. (Aspirin can promote bleeding, so you're better off with one of the other NSAIDs.)

### Vitamin and Mineral Supplements

In addition to a good multivitamin, there is evidence that particular vitamin and mineral supplements may help with menstrual problems.

- B vitamins: A number of studies have shown that taking at least 100 mg of vitamin $B_1$ (thiamine), and 100 mg of vitamin $B_6$, especially as part of a high-potency B-complex vitamin, can help with symptoms. (*Note:* Now Foods makes an excellent high-potency B-complex; each capsule includes 100 mg of $B_1$, $B_2$, $B_6$, $B_{12}$, and other essential vitamins and minerals.)
- Vitamin E: Vitamin E is thought to have antiprostaglandin properties, and 400 IU a day may help ease cramps, pain, and breast tenderness.
- Calcium: Taking 1,200 mg of calcium (combining diet and supplements) can help with water retention, cramps and back pain, and reduce overall severity of PMS symptoms after 3 months (and particularly if you add in some vitamin D). Don't forget that you can use chewable calcium carbonate such as Tums or Rolaids to count toward your 1,200 mg total. The calcium should be taken with 400 IU of vitamin D (*Note:* Most women get no more than half the recommended 1,200 mg of calcium per day.)

- Magnesium: Low levels of magnesium have been linked to PMS symptoms. Taking 200 to 400 mg per day of magnesium may help with various symptoms, including breast tenderness and bloating.
- Other vitamins: Vitamin A, C, and K are thought to help with clotting and circulation. A good multivitamin that contains these vitamins may be recommended.
- Iron supplements: For women with heavy bleeding, low iron levels, or even anemia, may occur. You should have blood tests to make sure you are iron-deficient before starting any iron supplements. Also, thyroid patients should allow at least 4 hours between taking thyroid hormone replacement drugs and taking any supplements with iron, as the iron can interfere with thyroid hormone absorption if taken too close to the thyroid medication.

### Essential Fatty Acids

Omega-3 and omega-6 fatty acids are polyunsaturated fats that the body cannot make itself, so they must be obtained from outside sources. Saturated fats, such as those found in red meat and butter, are associated with increased risk of disease, but the polyunsaturated essential fatty acids have positive health benefits. EFAs act as natural antiprostaglandins and anti-inflammatories, and may help with pain from inflammation, ease depression, and minimize breast pain and tenderness, among other health benefits.

Typically, we consume far more omega-6 fatty acids than omega-3, so many experts recommend supplementing the omega-3 intake.

Omega-3 fatty acids are found primarily in cold-water fish such as tuna, salmon, mackerel, herring, sardines, Atlantic halibut, and bluefish. While it's often recommended that you eat fish two to three times per week, there are also increasing calls to limit fish consumption to perhaps twice a week, because so many fish are contaminated with high levels of mercury. A good-quality, mercury-free fish oil supplement—I like Enzymatic Therapies Eskimo Oil—may help make up the difference. There are plant sources of omega-3 fatty acids as well. Canola oil, flaxseed and flaxseed oil, walnuts, and some leafy green vegetables are good sources of alpha-linolenic acid (ALA), a plant-based omega-3. For example, 1 ounce of walnuts supplies about 2 grams of plant-based omega-3 fatty acids, equivalent to the omega-3 in 3 ounces of salmon. Some foods have been enhanced. For example, Omega Eggs are enriched eggs.

Omega-6s are found in grains, many plant-based oils, poultry, and eggs. There are a number of therapeutic oils high in omega-6, including evening primrose oil (EPO), borage oil, and black currant seed oil. The omega-6 oils, and evening primrose oil in particular, have been found to calm inflammation, reduce breast tenderness, relieve bloating, and reduce cramps. To achieve antiprostaglandin benefits from EPO, 3 grams a day (3,000 mg) is recommended.

### Maca

Maca (*lepidium peruvianum chacon*) is also sometimes known as Peruvian ginseng, maca root, and maca-maca. It's a cruciferous vegetable that grows at high altitudes—between 12,500 and 14,500 feet—in the Andes. In addition to serving as a food source, the root of the plant has been used for several thousand years to enhance fertility, libido, and energy. Maca is an adaptogen, and seems to have its greatest effects on the reproductive and endocrine systems, including the ovaries, testes, adrenals, pancreas, and thyroid. Native practitioners and herbalists have traditionally recommended maca to help regulate and normalize menstrual cycles, enhance sex drive, and promote fertility.

According to Dr. Viana Muller, an anthropologist and herbalist with expertise in South American herbal medicine, "maca helps to normalize the menstrual cycle, both in terms of number of days in a cycle, the amount of blood flow, and the great reduction of pain and PMS."

## Herbs

- Red raspberry leaf tea (not raspberry tea) is considered an overall uterine tonic; it may help with heavy bleeding and reduce cramps and pain.
- Dong quai is generally known for helping overall uterine health and regulating the menstrual cycle. It may also relax the muscles of the uterus, helping to reduce menstrual cramps. Dong quai is available in many forms, including tinctures, pills, liquids, as a dried herb, and tea.
- Chasteberry, also known as chaste tree, chaste tree berry, vitex agnus-castus, or vitex, is the most recommended herb in Europe for PMS. The herb stimulates the pituitary to produce more luteinizing hormone, which then helps produce progesterone and lower prolactin. In that manner, chasteberry can help reduce various PMS symptoms by balancing the progesterone-estrogen ratio. It apparently can also help in regulating ovulation and in normalizing luteal phase length. It's often recommended to help bring on menstruation, reduce heavy periods, and reduce breast tenderness.

- Black cohosh is one of the most recommended herbs for women, used for everything from PMS and menstrual cramps to regulating menstrual cycles. It's thought that black cohosh reduces levels of luteinizing hormone and helps to regulate various symptoms.
- Cramp bark, in tea or pill form, is considered a uterine sedative, and is thought to help reduce menstrual cramp pain; it may also bring on delayed menstruation.
- Goldenrod, horsetail, hawthorn, and corn silk are herbal and natural diuretics that may help with bloating and water retention. I also particularly like a combination herbal formulation, Lean for Less Water Regulator, made by Health from the Sun, which includes several vitamins, iron, magnesium, and herbal diuretics, including lespedeza capitata powder, couch grass, java tea, and dandelion powder.
- Various herbs thought to be helpful for menorrhagia include yarrow, nettles, shepherd's purse, and marsh mallow.
- Kava, a natural tranquilizer, may help alleviate stress.
- Ginkgo biloba is reported to help reduce breast pain and tenderness.
- Saint-John's-wort may help alleviate mild depression in some people. (But it definitely should not be used if you are already taking prescription antidepressants.)

## The Soy Controversy

Practitioners often recommend that women take soy products, pills, protein powders, or soy foods in large quantities, because as a plant estrogen, soy can have some hormonal effects that may help with various symptoms.

The issue of soy is a controversial one. Some of the bioidentical hormones are actually derived from soy products, and appear to be effective in some people without side effects. And soy does have some health benefits, for example, helping to lower cholesterol. But overconsumption of soy has the potential to disrupt hormonal, reproductive, and endocrine function, according to some experts. At these higher levels, soy is no longer a food, but a drug, and the isoflavones act as endocrine-disrupting estrogens, with the potential to:

- Impair thyroid function
- Promote goiter
- Trigger autoimmune thyroid disease
- Increase the risk of developing thyroid cancer
- Impair fertility

At the levels many people think is healthy for diet, soy can prevent ovulation. According to researchers at the Soy Online Service, "as little as 30 grams (about 4 tablespoons) of soy per day can result in hypothyroidism."

According to the Weston Price Foundation, "60–100 mg isoflavones per day [is] an amount that provides the estrogen equivalent of the contraceptive pill."

In one study, premenopausal women were given 60 grams of soy protein per day for one month. Just one month on this regimen disrupted the menstrual cycle of most participants, and the effect continued for three months after soy in the diet was stopped. Another study found that intake of soy over a long period causes enlargement of the thyroid and suppresses thyroid function. Isoflavones at high levels can also negatively affect fertility.

Most natural practitioners I've consulted with tend to feel that if you are going to eat soy, limiting yourself to one serving a day is smart, and that some forms of soy are preferable to others. Soy in its fermented forms—tempeh, miso, and soy sauce—is safer than the unfermented forms, such as fresh soybeans (edamame), soy nuts, soy sprouts, soy milk and tofu, soy pills, powders, supplements, and soy protein powders.

## Other Treatments for Menstrual Disorders

### Acupuncture and Acupressure

Acupuncture and acupressure treatments have had some success in relieving menstrual distress, as well as improving mood due to better balance of brain chemicals. In one study, 43 patients were followed for a year; 90 percent of those who had acupuncture once a week through three menstrual cycles had less pain, and almost half used less pain medication during their menstrual cycles.

### Bright-Light Therapy

Some studies have suggested that bright-light therapy may also help with PMS symptoms. This is thought to have a beneficial effect on serotonin levels in the brain, which play an important role in regulating a person's mood. Bright-light therapy, which is used for seasonal affective disorder, involves sitting in front of a special bright light for several minutes to a half-hour each day, to help stimulate the brain chemicals. (A great resource for home bright-light therapy is a company called Sunbox, http://www.sunbox.com, 1-800-548-3968.)

### Heat Therapy

Heat can be a good treatment for pain during menstruation. Electric heating pads, warm baths, and even the portable charcoal-activated heating pads (i.e., ThermaCare heat wraps) may help with cramps and pain.

### Transcutaneous Electrical Nerve Stimulation

Some women find a treatment called transcutaneous electrical nerve stimulation (TENS) helpful for particular painful periods, or when they cannot use traditional pain relief medications. One study found that TENS relieved pain in as many as half of the people using the therapy, and another study found that it worked faster than the NSAID drug naproxen.

## Lifestyle Treatments

### Eating Habits

Changes to eating habits may help you deal with menstrual irregularities and symptoms.

- If menstrual problems are due to anorexia or consuming too few calories, eating habits may need to change in order for a normal menstrual cycle to resume.
- Consider a low-fat vegetarian diet. Some women find that it helps reduce the intensity and duration of painful periods and limits the duration of certain premenstrual symptoms such as mood, bloating, and water retention.

- Consider a low-fat diet. For some women, it can reduce estrogen levels, which can reduce the stimulation of the uterine liming, which helps minimize prostaglandins.
- Avoid salt, especially in the last few days before your period starts; this may help reduce bloating and fluid retention.
- Drink water, even more heavily in the week prior to your menstrual period, as water intake acts as a natural diuretic.
- Cut back on caffeine, to help reduce anxiety and irritability. Caffeine is also linked to breast pain and headaches. If it's too hard to go on and off caffeine, consider cutting it out completely.
- Cut out alcohol. Drinking alcohol before your period can make you feel more depressed.
- Stabilize blood sugar in the week before your period by eating smaller meals more frequently.
- Eat more oily fish in the week before and during menstruation; oily fish contain natural antiprostaglandins that can help relieve cramping and other symptoms.

### Exercise

Exercise is an essential part of dealing with menstrual irregularities, especially aerobic exercise, 30 minutes, four to six times a week if possible. Even a brisk walk can count. There are defenite benefits.

- Exercise helps release natural painkillers.
- Exercise suppresses the release of prostaglandins.
- Exercise helps reduce pelvic pain.
- Exercise helps with fatigue.
- Exercise helps relieve depression.

## Stress Management

Some experts have found that stress management can help with both the symptoms of menstrual irregularities and the actual irregularities themselves. It may seem improbable that stress could have an impact on the menstrual cycle, but recent studies in the field of psychoneuroimmunology show that the mind can communicate with the endocrine systems via cells called neurotransmitters.

You'll want to find the techniques that are most effective for you and learn to incorporate them into your regular activities. Here are some of the options.

- Relaxation
- Deep breathing or pranayama yoga breathing
- Yoga
- Tai chi
- Meditation
- Warm baths
- Listening to music
- Stretching
- Guided imagery and visualization
- Self-hypnosis
- Journaling
- Prayer
- Therapy, counseling, or support groups
- Creative therapies: art, music, and dance therapy

## Smoking Cessation

If you are a smoker experiencing menstrual problems, you have to stop smoking. Smoking is linked to so many issues, including longer bleeding, heavier bleeding, more pain during menstruation, and more variable cycles. And the more you smoke, the more likely you are to have more significant symptoms. Find what works, whether it's anti-anxiety medication, antidepressants, acupuncture, the nicotine patch, or a smoking cessation group—supplemented by exercise, stress reduction techniques, online support groups, and other tactics to help you quit.

### Sleep

Many women find that lack of sufficient sleep—and this means getting fever than eight hours of sleep a night—can aggravate cycle and flow irregularities, as well as menstrual pain. So, make a very basic lifestyle change—get at least eight hours of sleep a night.

## Sexual Dysfunction

According to a study reported in the February 1999 issue of the *Journal of the American Medical Association* (JAMA), about 43 percent of women suffer from chronic sexual dysfunction. This is thought to be an underestimate of the real level of sexual dysfunction in the United States. And these numbers are far exceeded by the 75 percent of us who are likely to experience shorter-term sexual problems at some point in our lives.

There are five different ways your sex life can suffer.

- *Avoidance*: Some people actively avoid sexual encounters completely, often due to some sort of trauma. The medical term is sexual aversion disorder.
- *Desire*: Problems with desire mean that you simply have no interest in sex, or you have less desire than you had

in the past. The medical term is hypoactive sexual desire disorder.

- *Arousal*: Problems with arousal mean that while you may want sex, your body does not become aroused or you cannot maintain arousal. The medical term for this problem is sexual arousal disorder.
- *Orgasm*: Orgasmic disorders mean that you are unable to have an orgasm. The medical term is orgasmic disorder.
- *Pain*: Problems with pain usually involve pain before, during, or after sex. This is known as dyspareunia. One of the most common causes of pain is vaginismus, which is an involuntary contraction of the muscles around the vagina in response to attempted penetration. Vaginismus can make sexual intercourse difficult or virtually impossible.

How many people with sexual dysfunction may actually have underlying thyroid disease that has not been diagnosed? It's not a question that has been studied, so numbers aren't available. It's clear, however, that for some people, a sexual problem—and in particular, a lack of desire or low libido— may be the first noticeable symptom of an underlying thyroid condition, a symptom that may resolve with proper diagnosis and optimized thyroid treatment.

Even among thyroid patients who are receiving optimal treatment, however, sexual dysfunction may be a continuing, unresolved problem. Many women still complain of a lack of sexual desire even after their doctors consider the thyroid problem sufficiently treated.

Kay describes her symptoms.

You got it right when you said *no* sex drive. Even though my thyroid levels are pretty good at the moment, my sex drive is basically nonexsistent and that stinks! My husband is a wonderful, attractive man who is the love of my life and I feel totally terrible when I say, "No, honey, not tonight" about 26 nights out of every month. He knows that it is my thyroid and the depression that goes with it that causes this, and he supports me totally, but I know he isn't happy about it.

Many doctors assume most sexual problems are psychological in origin. This is because we know that untreated depression, for example, can reduce sex drive. Besides depression, other psychological and emotional issues that affect your sex life include stress, anxiety, work or family responsibilities, worry over your sexual performance, relationship problems, boredom, unresolved sexual issues, past sexual trauma, poor body image, low self-esteem.

But some doctors now believe that, for the most part, sexual dysfunction is not a mental issue. Says Dr. Dana Ohk, a University of Michigan/Ann Arbor urologist: "We think that about 90 percent of sexual dysfunction actually has a physical basis."

Looking at the common physical causes, your doctor should rule out other conditions—in addition to thyroid problems—that can affect your sexual function. The most common culprits include diabetes, high blood pressure, heart disease, liver disease, kidney disease, pelvic injury, and neurological disorders. Alcohol or drug abuse—in particular, use of drugs such as cocaine and marijuana—should be discussed.

Your doctor should also review all medications and supplements you take, to ensure that you aren't taking anything that can affect sexual function. A number of drugs can cause sexual dysfunction. Perhaps the most common are the antidepressants. An estimated 40 percent of patients on antidepressants report problems with sexual function, in particular, the tricyclic antidepressants like clomipramine (Anafranil) and some SSRIs (Prozac, Paxil, Zoloft, and Lexapro). If you are being treated for depression, you may want to consider asking the doctor about bupoprion (Wellbutrin), an antidepressant not typically associated with sexual side effects.

Other drugs you'll want to discuss with your practitioner include:

- Antihistamines
- Anticancer drugs: tamoxifen and raloxifene, used to help prevent recurrent cancers
- Anticonvulsants: phenobarbital (Luminal), Dilantin, Mysloine, and Tegretol
- Antiandrogens: cimetidine and spironolactone
- Antihypertensives: blood pressure medications including alpha-blockers, beta-blockers (Inderal, Atenolol, Tenormin), diuretics, calcium channel blockers
- Antipsychotics: Thorazine, Haldol and Zyprexa
- Anti-anxiety medications: Xanax and Valium
- Birth control pills
- Chemotherapy drugs

There is also some evidence that appetite suppressants and opioid pain drugs may contribute to sexual dysfunction.

Your doctor may refer you to a sexual dysfunction specialist. Diagnostic tests for sexual function may be performed to assess the dysfunction. These can include:

- Measure of vaginal blood flow and engorgement, which can be measured by a tampon-shaped device in a process called vaginal photoplethysmography
- Vaginal pH testing, which can identify underlying infection and fluctuating hormone levels
- Pressure and temperature sensitivity testing, which measures the clitoris and labia's sensitivity to pressure and temperature via a device called a biothesiomater

Ultimately, though, for many thyroid patients, sexual dysfunction is a symptom of the overall hormonal imbalance, of which your thyroid is just a part. Sexual function and our hormones are intricately related. For example, during the menstrual cycle, sex drive fluctuates, with the highest levels often reported around ovulation. That's Mother Nature's way of encouraging reproduction. After pregnancy and childbirth, and during breastfeeding, hormonal shifts often reduce your sexual desire—again, Mother Nature's way of protecting the baby and ensuring his or her survival. And the period after menopause, when estrogen levels drop, can reduce sex drive, as well as cause vaginal dryness and pain that make sexual intercourse uncomfortable. Imbalances in estrogen, progesterone, and testosterone all can negatively affect sexual function.

Your doctor, therefore, needs to pay particular attention to hormone levels and balance. This means that, in addition to your thyroid, your doctor should evaluate estrogen levels, testosterone, and progesterone, plus DHEA. Adrenal function should also be checked, particularly if the testosterone levels turn out to be low.

## Treatments

In addition to the most basic—thyroid evaluation and diagnosis, followed by optimal thyroid treatment—the most important thing you can do to help restore normal sexual function may well be overall hormonal balancing, as described in Chapter 11.

For some people, however, a more targeted hormonal approach may help. This might include:

- Testosterone, which for women is available as a prescription pill or capsule and as a prescription testosterone propionate cream.
- Low-dose nonconjugated prescription estrogen capsules, patches, gel, or cream
- Prescription progesterone capsules
- Nonprescription progesterone cream or gels

*Note*: Be careful about soy-based supplements and food products that are supposed to act "like" estrogen for menopause relief. Many of these products contain levels of soy isoflavones that can worsen hypothyroidism in some women.

You may also wish to investigate supplements that may help with various aspects of sexual function. Supplements can have various—and sometimes serious—side effects, so you shouldn't self-treat. Talk to your practitioner regarding these products. Some supplements that may help increase sex drive and energy include:

- Arginine: an amino acid
- Ashwaganda: an Indian Ayurvedic herb

- Asian ginseng (panax): which can reportedly help sexual energy increase
- Avena-sativa or oat extract (Vigorex): reportedly helps with sex drive
- Damiana: an aphrodisiac herb from Mexico thought to stimulate production of testosterone in women
- DHEA (dehydroepiandrosterone): a precursor hormone that converts to testosterone in the body
- Horny goat weed: used by Chinese herbalists to improve sexual functions in both men and women
- Maca: a South American herbal supplement that can help women with libido
- Kava kava: an herb most known for use in relaxation but can also be useful as an aphrodisiac for women
- Zinc: low levels have been associated with low sex drive

In addition to supplements taken internally, there are external vaginal creams and lubricants that can help with dryness, and, in some cases, help with sexual stimulation as well.

## Other Helpful Approaches

An important thing that you can do to help sexual dysfunction is to lose weight. Excess weight can affect your self-image—making you feel less sexy and less interested in sex. And, medically, being overweight can reduce libido. Some experts believe that a ten- to twenty-pound weight loss in an overweight woman can substantially reduce levels of sex hormone–binding globulin (SHBG), which then frees up estrogen and testosterone, allowing them to get back to their regular functions in your reproductive system.

Exercise is also essential, as it helps improve blood flow to all body parts. Research has found that people who exercise regularly have higher levels of desire, greater sexual confidence and frequency, and an enhanced ability to be aroused and achieve orgasm—no matter what their age. The best type of exercise is aerobic exercise, because it can trigger the release of endorphins, chemicals in the brain that create a feeling of well-being. But all exercise can help, and as you become slimmer, stronger, or more toned, you're likely to enjoy a more positive body image, which can also contribute to improved sexual function.

When there are other psychological and self-esteem issues blocking healthy sexual desire, therapy can sometimes help. Traditional psychotherapy may help identify and resolve root causes of problems, improve self-esteem, or teach new skills in self-expression. Communications or couples counseling may help improve the relationship. Sex therapy may help resolve specific dysfunctions and teach techniques that aid in sexual desire and satisfaction. The American Association of Sex Educators, Counselors, and Therapists can help you find a qualified therapist.

## Chapter 7

# Pregnancy Challenges

A baby is God's opinion that life should go on.

—Carl Sandburg

Pregnancy can be a challenging time for women who have preexisting thyroid conditions. A woman with thyroid disease must prepare carefully for pregnancy, and be monitored and treated appropriately throughout the pregnancy in order to ensure her health, the continuation of her pregnancy, and the health of her baby.

Pregnancy is also when thyroid problems may appear for the first time in many women. Because thyroid conditions can have a negative impact on your health and the health of your unborn baby, the viability of the pregnancy, and even the physical and intellectual development of the baby, it is critical that thyroid problems be diagnosed and treated promptly and correctly during pregnancy.

Diagnosing and managing thyroid disease during pregnancy can be a challenge, however, because the symptoms of thyroid disease are similar to many common pregnancy symptoms. For example, in pregnancy, many women experience an increase in metabolism, with difficulty sleeping, increased heart rate, and palpitations. These symptoms can be the same in hyperthyroidism. At the same time, fatigue, hair loss, and weight gain are also normal pregnancy symptoms, yet can also be symptoms of hypothyroidism.

This chapter discusses how women with a diagnosed thyroid condition should prepare for pregnancy, and how they should cope with the onset of various thyroid problems during pregnancy in order to ensure the best possible outcome for themselves and the baby.

## Pregnancy and the Thyroid

The thyroid goes through a number of important changes during pregnancy, and proper thyroid function and hormonal balance is essential to a healthy pregnancy and healthy baby.

### TBG Increases

In pregnancy, there is an increase in production of T4-binding globulin, known as TBG. TBG is a protein that acts as a transporter for thyroid hormone in the bloodstream. This TBG increase sets off a chain of events that affect the overall hormonal picture in pregnancy:

- The estrogens can stimulate the development of TBG development; as estrogen levels rise in pregnancy, TBG levels rise as well, in some cases nearly doubling.

- The TBG actually binds to thyroxine (T4) in the bloodstream, which lowers the free T4 levels.
- The brain perceives the lowered free T4 levels as being insufficient (hypothyroidism), and so TSH elevates.
- The elevated TSH triggers the thyroid to produce more thyroid hormone.
- T4 and T3 levels increase

This process is important, because there is an increased need for thyroid hormone during pregnancy, in particular, early pregnancy when the baby does not have a functional thyroid and relies on the mother's extra production for all its thyroid hormonal needs.

### Need for Increased Iodine

Pregnancy creates a need for increased levels of iodine for the mother. Iodine is the building block of thyroid hormone, and the need to produce increased thyroid hormone means that more iodine must be readily available from the beginning of pregnancy in order to meet that need.

If the mother does not have a sufficient iodine level, both she and her baby can end up hypothyroid. Severe iodine deficiency in pregnancy can have serious consequences for the child, resulting in cretinism, mental retardation, and deafness. Even minor iodine deficiency in a mother can reduce IQ levels and affect cognitive development in her baby.

In order to avoid this problem, women need sufficient iodine levels before becoming pregnant. Typically they need supplementation during the first and second trimesters. Many experts recommend iodine intake (food plus supplements) of at least 200 mcg/day prior to conception and during the pregnancy.

## Hyperthyroid Effects of HCG

The HCG released during pregnancy stimulates the thyroid. HCG levels rise, and reach their highest point typically at the end of the first trimester, around 13 weeks. Because the thyroid is stimulated, TSH may even be suppressed to hyperthyroid levels, but typically, this does not require treatment and resolves later in the pregnancy.

# General Preparation for Pregnancy

Before becoming pregnant, you definitely want to make sure you're eating habits are as healthy as possible. Eat lots of vegetables, fruits, low-fat proteins, high-fiber grains. Avoid pesticides and hormones in meats, dairy, and produce as much as possible. Limit your caffeine intake, and if you drink alcohol, do so moderately.

You should also stop smoking. Smoking can be harmful to an unborn baby, and it also has a negative impact on your thyroid function; it can impair fertility and affect your health during pregnancy.

Also, discuss any drugs you take regularly with your doctor, as you may need to taper off some prescription medications before trying to become pregnant. (Keep in mind, however, that thyroid hormone replacement must always be taken throughout pregnancy.)

You should also start a good prenatal vitamin for several months prior to getting pregnant and throughout the pregnancy. If you are hypothyroid and taking thyroid hormone replacement, do keep in mind that iron interferes with the absorption of thyroid hormone, so you should *not* take your prenatal vitamin with iron within three to four hours of taking your thyroid medication. Taking them at separate times of the day allows you to get full absorption of the thyroid hormone without interference from the iron. Calcium supplements, which some pregnant women take, also need to be taken with care by thyroid patients, since calcium can also block the absorption of thyroid hormone. It's advisable to wait two to three hours before or after taking your thyroid medication to take your calcium. The same guidelines should be followed for calcium-fortified foods as well, such as orange juice with calcium.

*All* women—not just ones with a thyroid condition—who are getting ready to conceive should take a folic acid supplement for several months before attempting conception. Since folic acid plays a key role in early cell and tissue formation, as well as the production of DNA, it's important to have a ready store of folic acid in the body both before and during pregnancy. Neural-tube defects typically appear in the growing fetus at four weeks of age, long before many women even know they're pregnant, which is why you need to start taking folic acid before you even try to get pregnant.

Studies have shown that numerous birth defects, such as spina bifida, anencephaly, and other neural-tube defects, have been linked to low levels of folic acid in pregnant women. According to the Centers for Disease Control, anywhere from 50 to 70 percent of some neural-tube defects could have been prevented if the mothers had had an adequate supply of folic acid. Folic acid is a B vitamin often found in green leafy vegetables, dried legumes, fruits, and orange juice from concentrate. It's also found in some fortified cereals. Both the CDC and the March of Dimes recommend that women take 400 micrograms (0.4 mg) of synthetic folic acid every day, as well as eating a healthy, balanced diet. You should be able to find synthetic folic acid supplements in your local grocery store, drugstore, or online.

# Preparing for Pregnancy
# If You're Already Hypothyroid

Most women with thyroid conditions end up hypothyroid. The end result for most women with Graves' disease or hyperthyroidism is radioactive iodine, which disables the thyroid and makes you hypothyroid. Women with thyroid cancer, goiter, or nodules often end up having the thyroid removed surgically, which makes them hypothyroid. And many women are hypothyroid due to Hashimoto's disease or for other reasons.

When you're hypothyroid, you may be concerned that pregnancy is going to be particularly difficult for you. You are right to acknowledge that a healthy pregnancy will require some extra planning and effort on your part, but generally, women who are informed, prepared, have a knowledgeable doctor, and whose thyroid condition is properly managed and treated should be able to go through pregnancy without any significant difficulties.

## *Optimize Your Thyroid Level for Maximum Fertility*

One of the most important things you can do is to optimize your thyroid levels before you try to become pregnant. Not only is it helpful to ensure a good outcome for the pregnancy, but it may actually be necessary for you simply to become pregnant.

Most doctors use the TSH level as a gauge. What's the optimal TSH level in order to become pregnant and maintain a successful pregnancy for both mother and baby? That's a difficult question, because different doctors have different answers. Some women may have been told that their TSH level is "normal," and they shouldn't have any trouble getting pregnant, yet they suffer years of "unexplained" infertility. Others may be told to not even attempt conceiving until the thyroid levels stabilize in the TSH range of 1.0 to 2.0.

Part of the source of the confusion stems from the definition of normal, and much of it depends on what numbers the laboratory considers high, normal, and low.

While it's a relief to be told your thyroid is normal, the term *normal* is no help. Insist on getting the exact number, along with the normal range for your lab. At many labs in North America, the normal range is somewhere around 0.5 to 5.5 (over 5.5 is hypothyroid/underactive, and under 0.5 is hyperthyroid/overactive). In 2003, however, the American Association of Clinical Endocrinologists, along with various physicians who make laboratory standards, recommended new laboratory guidelines of 0.3 to 3.0. These doctors believe that levels above 3.0 should be considered hypothyroid.

At Endo 2005, the Endocrine Society's annual meeting, held in San Diego, research was presented that looked at the body's response to the increased demand that pregnancy puts on the mother's thyroid production. According to the researchers, nonpregnant reference ranges are "unreliable for assessing thyroid status during pregnancy." The researchers concluded the following:

> There is growing consensus that a first trimester serum TSH above 2.5 mIU/L may indicate thyroxine insufficiency, especially if TPOAb [thyroid peroxidase antibodies] is detected.

According to new research just published in early 2006, during a normal pregnancy, the following are the TSH normal ranges for iodine-sufficient women who do not have autoimmune antibodies:

- First trimester: 0.24–2.99
- Second trimester: 0.46–2.95
- Third trimester: 0.43–2.78

Some experts now believe that if TSH is above 2.0 in early gestation, hypothyroidism treatment should be considered. There has been a suggestion that while there is not yet sufficient evidence for the benefits of treating pregnant women with subclinical hypothyroidism, there are enough arguments that strongly suggest that since it's not dangerous, levothyroxine treatment may be beneficial for both mother and baby.

When I started doing my preconception workup in 1996, my TSH level at the time was 4.1, in an overall TSH normal range of .5 to 5.5. I was feeling okay—not perfect, but pretty well—and thought because I was in the normal range, this would be a good time to finally try to get pregnant. My endocrinologist (a woman with more than 20 years treating women with thyroid problems and thyroid-related infertility) believed firmly at that time that women needed to be maintained at a TSH level between 1 and 2 (which was considered low by some doctors) and that a woman with evidence of thyroid disease needed to be in that same range in order to get pregnant and maintain the pregnancy.

Interestingly, there is other research that backs up this theory. A study reported on in 1994 in the *Journal of Clinical Endocrinology and Metabolism* looked at pregnant women with thyroid antibodies and TSH in the normal range. The study found that women with autoimmune thyroid disease had TSH values significantly higher, though still normal, in the first trimester than in women with healthy pregnancies used as controls. The higher TSH level of the women with autoimmune thyroid disease? 1.6. The normal TSH level for the control group of pregnant woman without autoimmune thyroid disease? 0.9. A TSH of 0.9 is a far cry from the so-called normal TSH levels of 3 or 4 or 5 that some doctors have felt are no impediment whatsoever to getting—or staying—pregnant.

## Get Enough Iodine

Iodine is particularly important for thyroid health, and proper iodine intake is even more essential during pregnancy. Until recently, it was assumed that iodine deficiency is not a particular problem in the United States, Japan, and some European countries, where iodine supplementation programs have been in place for many years. Recently, however, studies have shown that iodine intake has dropped significantly in the United States, and as many as 15 percent of women of childbearing age and almost 7 percent of pregnant women were iodine-deficient.

Mild iodine deficiency during pregnancy can contribute to hypothyroidism in the mother, and various issues in the child, including reduced IQ. Significant iodine deficiency during pregnancy—which is seen in some countries that do not have routine iodine supplementation—can cause significant thyroid enlargement (goiter) in the mother, and major birth defects and even cretinism in the child.

Typically, women should supplement with approximately 150 mcg a day of iodine for several months before they become pregnant. It takes two to three months at minimum to reach a state where the stored iodine is sufficient to meet the needs of pregnancy.

## Confirm Your Pregnancy Early

Try to make sure that you find out you are pregnant as early as possible. One way is to use a home pregnancy test kit. Some kits (I like the E.P.T. kits) are sensitive as early as 10 days post conception. You should not wait for a missed period in order to confirm your pregnancy. I suggest you test as early as possible, because the earlier you confirm the pregnancy, the earlier you can start taking the best possible care of yourself, increasingly your thyroid dosage as recommended by your doctor, setting up appointments with your practitioners, and ensuring that your hypothyroidism is properly monitored and treated.

Studies have confirmed that the levothyroxine requirements in most women with preexisting hypothyroidism must be increased during pregnancy. The July 15, 2004, issue of the *New England Journal of Medicine* reported on a study conducted at Brigham and Women's Hospital in Boston. That study found that 85 percent of pregnant women with hypothyroidism require an increase in thyroid hormone replacement drug to protect the baby, and most needed as much as a 47 percent increase in dose at around eight weeks into the pregnancy.

The body's increased demand for levothyroxine during pregnancy was seen as early as the fifth week of gestation, leading the researchers to recommend that women themselves raise their thyroid drug intake immediately upon confirming pregnancy. According to the study authors,

> We suggest that women with hypothyroidism be instructed to increase their usual levothyroxine intake by two additional doses each week immediately on confirmation of pregnancy and to contact their health care provider so that a program of test-guided dose adjustments can be instituted.

You should discuss this approach with your practitioner before you try to get pregnant, so that you have a physician-directed plan for your treatment for the time between when you confirm the pregnancy with a home test and have your thyroid function evaluated by the doctor.

You'll definitely want thyroid tests as soon as possible after you know you're pregnant; at 8 to 12 weeks; at 20 weeks; and again later in the third trimester, because your need for increased thyroid hormone may not show up until later in the pregnancy.

Keep in mind that if you do not have residual thyroid tissue (after RAI for thyrotoxicosis or surgery for cancer) you are likely to require a larger increase in levothyroxine, while women with residual functional thyroid tissue (Hashimoto's) typically require a smaller dosage increase. Women who have had RAI for hyperthyroidism show the greatest need for increased dosage—a mean increase of 46 percent, according to one study. As many as 25 percent of those women who begin pregnancy with a normal TSH level in the first trimester, and 37 percent of those with normal TSH levels in the second trimester, will require dosage increase later in the pregnancy.

What you do not want to do is to get pregnant, continue taking the same dose of thyroid hormone as always, call to see an obstetrician, and be told that your first appointment will be when you are 9 or 10 weeks pregnant. This can endanger your pregnancy. There are a number of medical and hormonal reasons why your thyroid hormone requirements go up so dramatically in early pregnancy, but the most important one is that your baby's thyroid health depends completely on you. In the first trimester, your baby develops arms, legs, a beating heart, and a brain, but an as-yet nonworking, but fully formed thyroid gland. The fetus needs a steady, appropriate supply of hormones to ensure proper development, and the only place to get it is from the mother. If it's not readily available, the fetus's development can suffer. If you wait until you are 8 or 9 weeks postconception, you can compromise your baby's health and development.

When I became pregnant in the spring of 1997, I tested positive via home pregnancy test only nine days postconception. This is fairly unusual: some women who are pregnant don't test positive until around 14 days postconception or later. I had a blood test a few days later to confirm the pregnancy at my regular doctor's office. I knew officially I was pregnant at only three weeks, which is when I called to schedule my first obstetrician (ob-gyn) appointment. My ob-gyn wanted to schedule me to come in sometime in the eighth or ninth week. I insisted on scheduling the first visit as soon as they could fit me in, which was two weeks. When I went in to the obstetrician, I asked for a TSH test. Interestingly, just five weeks after conception, my TSH had already gone up to 3, from 1.2. In keeping with my endocrinologist's directions to keep my levels below 2, my dosage was upped slightly, I was retested two weeks later, and my TSH returned to around 1.4.

The first thing you should do if you suspect or know you're pregnant is call your doctor's office and push to be seen as early as possible. Some doctors don't like to see pregnant patients until well into the first trimester. For some women, this is fine, but as a patient with a thyroid condition, it's absolutely vital that you start the process of monitoring thyroid hormones and antibody levels as soon as possible.

Hopefully, you have been taking a prenatal vitamin all along, but if not, start immediately. Just make sure to take it appropriately: at the same time every day and at least three to four hours apart from your thyroid medication so that the iron doesn't interfere with the absorption of your thyroid hormones.

## Prepare for Your First Doctor Visit

Usually when you are pregnant, most of your medical treatment transfers over to an obstetrician during this period. Here are some questions to ask your obstetrician.

- Have you treated many people with thyroid conditions before, and what was the outcome?
- How soon, and how often, will I receive regular monitoring of my thyroid hormone and antibodies?
- What levels of T3, T4, and antibodies do you consider normal for a successful pregnancy?
- Can I stay on my regular thyroid treatment regimen, or do you propose a change? If so, why?
- Will I be considered a high-risk pregnancy?

If you feel that you aren't getting satisfactory answers, you're getting the brush-off, or the doctor simply doesn't have much information about how to manage thyroid disease in pregnancy, you may want to add an endocrinologist to your medical team or find an obstetrician with expertise managing high-risk thyroid patients. You and your baby are far too important to settle for less.

At the first prenatal checkup, your doctor will likely take a complete medical history (assuming he or she did not do one at a preconception workup) involving such things as past pregnancies and their outcomes, familial history of diseases and problems, medications you currently take, and the like. At this visit—or possibly beforehand, so you can discuss the results with the doctor—you should ask for a complete thyroid panel, so he or she can review your hormone levels and evaluate whether they are adequate enough to sustain a healthy pregnancy.

# Preparing for Pregnancy If You're Hyperthyroid or Have Graves' Disease

If you are hyperthyroid or have Graves' disease, many doctors will advise that you not get pregnant unless the condition is either permanently treated with radioactive iodine (RAI) or surgery or you have a mild condition that is well controlled with antithyroid drugs.

The concern, however, is that, due to the immunologic and hormonal changes of pregnancy, even mild hyperthyroidism can escalate to more serious hyperthyroidism, including high blood pressure and high heart rate, that could endanger the health of both mother and baby.

This is why an irreversible, permanent treatment like RAI or surgery is preferred, as the woman will then become hypothyroid for life, which is considered by physicians to be easier to monitor and treat than hyperthyroidism.

If you have thyroid surgery, you become hypothyroid, and you should get stabilized on thyroid hormone replacement drugs when you become pregnant. (See the previous section on preparing for pregnancy if you're hypothyroid.)

If you've had RAI, most doctors recommend waiting and getting your thyroid hormone replacement regimen stabilized before getting pregnant, to reduce any potential risk of radioactivity to your baby. How long you should wait depends on the expert—recommendations range from three months to a year. The consensus in the United States is that you should wait at least six months. (You should, therefore, also use reliable birth control during this period. It's particularly important because in some women, fertility may be increased after hyperthyroidism starts to resolve.) If you are hyperthyroid and want to get pregnant quickly, surgery may be the best option.

Even if you have been treated for Graves' disease with either RAI or surgery, if you are planning to become pregnant, you should know that you may still have a high reading of thyroid antibodies in your bloodstream. You should have antibody testing prior to becoming pregnant; some doctors recommend a course of antithyroid drugs to bring your level of antibodies to a normal, manageable level before pregnancy.

If you have had RAI or surgery for Graves' disease or hyperthyroidism, your baby still has a risk of fetal and neonatal hyperthyroidism. The risk, however, depends in your levels of thyrotropin-receptor antibodies during pregnancy. You'll want to have these antibodies measured early in the pregnancy in order to evaluate the risk to your baby.

If you are being treated for hyperthyroidism with antithyroid drugs and then become pregnant, be sure to talk to your doctor. If you are taking methimazole, it's likely that your doctor will consider switching you to PTU, because it's safer for your unborn baby. And, if you are already taking PTU, it's likely your dosage will change, so be sure to advise your physician as soon as possible of your pregnancy.

## Managing Hypothyroidism That Develops During Pregnancy

For some women, hypothyroidism first appears during pregnancy. An underactive thyroid can endanger the mother's health during pregnancy, and puts the pregnancy—as well as the baby's future health—at risk as well.

According to the AACE, 1 in 50 women in the United States will be diagnosed with hypothyroidism during pregnancy.

Although it is known that thyroid hormone is needed for the developing fetal brain, scientists have yet to pinpoint exactly how maternal thyroid hormone interacts with fetal development. We do know, however that fetal development is highly dependent on the mother's thyroid hormone levels: during the first trimester, the fetus is totally dependent on the mother's thyroid function; during the second trimester, the fetus is partially dependent on the mother's supply of thyroid hormones.

Maternal hypothyroidism, particularly during the first and second trimesters, may endanger the pregnancy itself or, if the pregnancy continues, result in irreversible damage to the baby.

For example, a report in the *Journal of Medical Screening* showed that pregnant hypothyroid women who were not receiving treatment had nearly four times the risk of a late miscarriage (second trimester or later) than other women.

One study showed the following pregnancy-related concerns among pregnant women with either overt or subclinical (low-level) hypothyroidism.

- 21 percent of the overtly hypothyroid and 15 percent of subclinically hypothyroid had pregnancy-induced hypertension.
- 6.6 percent of the overtly hypothyroid and 3.5 percent of the subclinically hypothyroid had postpartum hemorrhage.
- 5 percent of the overtly hypothyroid mothers had placenta abruptio.

The danger to the baby is also evident.

- 6.6 percent of the overtly hypothyroid and 1.7 percent of the subclinically hypothyroid mothers delivered stillborn babies.
- 3.3 percent of the overtly hypothyroid mothers had newborns with congenital malformations.

- 16.6 percent of the overtly hypothyroid and 8.7 percent of the subclinically hypothyroid had low-birth-weight newborns.

One of the most well-known concerns is that in order for the fetal brain to develop properly, an adequate supply of thyroid hormone is vital. Lack of such hormones—as may occur in women who haven't been treated for their underactive thyroid—can cause negative effects on the baby, including lower IQ and possible learning problems. In an oft-repeated 1999 study reported in the *New England Journal of Medicine*, children born to mothers whose hypothyroidism was not being treated scored several points lower on an IQ test that children of nonthyroid patients. The study went on to note, however, that children whose mothers were undergoing treatment for an underactive thyroid scored almost the same as children born to mothers with normal thyroid function.

## Symptoms

Symptoms of hypothyroidism in pregnancy can be very similar to those of pregnancy, so it can be more difficult for a woman and her doctor to pinpoint. Common symptoms include:

- Fatigue and lethargy
- Constipation
- Intolerance to cold
- Depression, moodiness
- Stiffness, cramps in muscles, body aches and pains
- Dry, brittle hair and skin
- Hair loss
- Memory problems
- Goiter or enlarged neck

- Swelling in feet and hands
- Puffiness in the face and eyes

If you are having these symptoms, don't let your doctor just dismiss it as "normal pregnancy symptoms." Insist on having your thyroid tested.

Jane went through three pregnancies experiencing a host of symptoms.

My pregnancy was going extremely well until the seventh month. I gained a total of 26 pounds in one month and my ob/gyn just told me to "lay off the salt and sugar" and you will notice less weight gain. At five feet, four and a half inches and 93 pounds just seven months previous, I had no idea that pregnancy could change a body so drastically. I got increasingly fatigued day by day and my face broke out terribly. I had never had acne in my life. After delivery, some of my symptoms faded, but some lingered. I was able to lose the entire 82 pounds I gained during the pregnancy. My hair stopped falling out in globs and the panic attacks seemed to dissipate. The fatigue and menstrual cramps still gave me problems. I noticed that I craved more and more sleep; the more I got, the more I wanted. When I did get sleep, nothing could wake me. Not shouting, not alarm clocks, nothing. Upon waking, I felt I was in a drunken stupor for the first two hours and began drinking coffee like mad. After my second pregnancy, my menstrual cycle began and stopped at crazy intervals; some months I would have two in one month, some months I would not have one at all. I had high cholesterol. That was alarming to me because I only eat white meat of chicken or turkey and steered clear of fatty foods. After my third pregnancy, I felt as though I was slowly dying.

Only after the third pregnancy was she diagnosed with an underactive thyroid condition.

## Diagnosis

To identify hypothyroidism, your doctor will typically do a TSH test. Even mild deficiency in thyroid during early pregnancy can potentially have a negative impact on both mother and baby, so researchers have been focusing more attention on what the optimal levels should be during pregnancy. In a study presented at the 13th International Thyroid Congress, in Buenos Aires in 2005, researchers reported on an assessment of pregnant women. They indicated that in the first trimester, TSH should not be above 2.5, as that level suggests thyroid deficiency. This is particularly true if thyroid peroxidase antibodies are detected, so you may wish to ask your practitioner to also do antibody testing.

Keep in mind that you should have your doctor check not only TSH and antibodies, but also free T4 levels. According to research presented at the June 2000 Endocrine Society conference, there is increasing evidence that even normal free T4 levels that fall into the lowest 10th percentile during the early stages of pregnancy can be associated with poor infant development.

Low-normal free T4 is not defined as maternal hypothyroidism when TSH is normal, but these outcomes indicate that screening and treatment for thyroid problems may be warranted in all women. The study concluded that women with a low-normal free T4—in the lowest 10th percentile at 12 weeks gestation—are at risk for children with developmental delay. Further, the researchers found that "TSH, during early gestation, seems to be without any value to pick up these women at risk." So, you may wish to consult with a cutting-edge endocrinologist or thyroid expert who is willing to monitor not only your TSH but your free T4 levels throughout your pregnancy.

## Treatment

If you are diagnosed as being hypothyroid while you are pregnant, you need to treat your diagnosis seriously and take action as early as possible. Your doctor will prescribe a natural or synthetic thyroid hormone replacement for you to take daily, and you need to take it properly. You will also need to have your thyroid levels monitored regularly, to ensure that your dosage is correct, as fluctuating hormone levels during pregnancy can affect your thyroid hormone needs.

In newly diagnosed hypothyroid pregnant women, experts recommend that the full replacement dose be started immediately. They suggest that two to three times the daily dose may be prescribed for two to three days to help rapidly normalize the thyroid function.

*Important Note*: Over the last few decades, women have become more aware of the cautions against use of prescription and nonprescription drugs during pregnancy. While these cautions are typically warranted, this warning should *never* apply to hypothyroidism. Your thyroid medication, such as Synthroid, Levoxyl, Levothroid, Armour, Thyrolar, etc., is safe to take during pregnancy, and in fact you could be doing your baby much more harm—irreparable brain damage, for instance—if you *don't* take your prescribed thyroid drugs. Just as an insulin-dependent diabetic cannot stop taking insulin during pregnancy, a woman who is hypothyroid should not stop taking her thyroid hormone drugs.

It's also important that you take your thyroid hormone properly, in order to get maximum benefit:

- Always check the prescription against what you receive. Don't allow generic substitutions.
- Most doctors feel that taking thyroid hormone on an empty stomach allows for maximum absorption. If you can, take your thyroid medicine first thing in the morning, at least an hour before eating, to allow for maximum absorption.
- If you start or stop eating high-fiber foods, get your thyroid rechecked, because it may change your absorption of thyroid medicines.
- Take vitamins or supplements with iron, including prenatal vitamins, at least two to three hours apart from your thyroid hormone. Iron can interfere with thyroid hormone absorption.
- Do not take calcium and calcium-fortified orange juice within two to three hours of taking thyroid hormone.
- Many pregnant women take antacids, during pregnancy. Don't take antacids within two to three hours of your thyroid hormone. Antacids contain calcium.
- Consistency is vital to your success. If nausea prevents you from taking your pills on an empty stomach, you should take your thyroid pill every day with food, rather than miss taking it or taking it erratically, some days with food, some days without. You may stabilize at a slightly higher dosage than if you weren't taking your pill with food, but you'll get to the right dosage.

Many guidelines say that in addition to being tested as soon as you confirm the pregnancy, and again during the first trimester, you should also have your thyroid function checked at least once during each subsequent trimester.

### A Personal Note

My main concern going through pregnancy with hypothyroidism? More weight gain that I'd have liked, which led to a borderline blood sugar problem that the doctor said wasn't gestational diabetes, but was close to it, late in the pregnancy. I ate very healthily—I thought—but looking back, I realize my diet was very heavy in carbohydrates and fruits. I think that hypothyroidism's tendency to give some people an exaggerated insulin response and near-diabetic blood sugar levels may make some pregnant women with hypothyroidism more susceptible to greater weight gain, and borderline or full-blown gestational diabetes. If I have another baby, I would ask for a consult with a nutritionist to devise a low-glycemic diet that would provide sufficient nourishment for me and the baby, but would balance blood sugar, and minimize unnecessarily weight gain. Luckily, I had a pretty uneventful pregnancy and an easy Cesarean section (my baby was breech, and there is a slightly increased risk of breech delivery in hypothyroid mothers) and my daughter was born a healthy 8½ pounds.

## Hashimoto's Disease

If you are pregnant and have been told you have Hashimoto's disease, you're not alone. Hashimoto's is the most common cause of hypothyroidism for pregnant women in this country. The elevated thyroid autoantibody levels—a distinguishing characteristic of autoimmune thyroid disease—are the biggest concern for pregnant women. Left untreated, the autoantibodies can spiral out of control, thereby attacking the fetus as a foreign invader.

Autoimmune disease and elevated antibodies are linked to fertility and pregnancy-related problems. For example, several studies have indicated that women with Hashimoto's disease are two to five times more likely to suffer fetal loss in the first 12 weeks of pregnancy, as opposed to women without thyroid autoimmunity. The issue of antibodies and their impact on fertility is discussed in Chapter 8.

You may worry that if you have Hashimoto's, your baby will too. It's rare, but it can happen. However, since Hashimoto's typically doesn't appear until the second decade of life, it's not likely to be seen in infants. Congenital hypothyroidism appears in 1 in 4,000 or 5,000 newborns. If thyroid therapy is started during their first three months, most of these children will have normal intellectual development. Untreated, however, their hypothyroidism can lead to serious mental and physical impairment. In the United States, all newborns are required to be tested for low T4 levels; the test is typically done along with the heel stick for phenylketonuria (PKU). But you may want to just double-check at the hospital or with your pediatrician at your first postnatal visit, to ensure that the thyroid test was performed.

## Graves' Disease, Hyperthyroidism, and Pregnancy

Graves' disease in pregnancy is not very common—only about 1 in 500 women develop it during pregnancy. Another form of hyperthyroidism, known as gestational transient thyrotoxicosis (GTT), is more common, occurring in as many as 2 to 3 out of every 100 pregnancies. While Graves' disease can be serious during pregnancy, GTT is considered milder.

Uncontrolled hyperthyroidism, especially during the second half of pregnancy, can lead to a variety of serious—even fatal, in rare cases—consequences for both the you and your baby. It's absolutely vital to take a diagnosis of hyperthyroidism quite seriously and follow your doctor's guidance.

When hyperthyroidism is not treated during pregnancy, you are at higher risk of a number of complications, including heart problems, high blood pressure, extreme morning sickness, pre-eclampsia, congestive heart failure, and even a life-threatening condition known as thyroid storm, where heart rate and blood pressure become uncontrollably high. Thyroid storm can be triggered by labor and delivery in a woman with untreated hyperthyroidism.

The risk to your baby is also significant, as untreated hyperthyroidism in a mother can cause several complications.

- Miscarriage
- Pre-eclampsia
- Placental abruption
- Intrauterine growth retardation
- Premature labor and delivery
- Low birth weight
- Stillbirth
- Fetal or neonatal hyperthyroidism

### Symptoms

The symptoms of hyperthyroidism in pregnancy may be hard to identify, because they are similar to those of pregnancy itself. Fatigue, anxiety, insomnia—all common symptoms of pregnancy—are also symptoms of hyperthyroidism.

Neck enlargement (goiter) is seen in almost all pregnant women with Graves' disease and hyperthyroidism; the gland is usually two to four times larger than its normal size. These are other common symptoms.

- Failure to gain weight or weight loss
- Pulse rate over 100
- Heart palpitations
- Arrhythmias or atrial fibrillation
- Higher blood pressure
- Difficulty concentrating
- Excessive nausea and vomiting
- Nervousness, anxiety, restlessness, fidgety behavior
- Depression, moodiness
- Tremor
- Intolerance to heat, excessive sweating
- Diarrhea
- Arm and leg muscle pain or weakness
- Difficulty climbing stairs
- A stare or protrusion of the eyes
- Vision problems: blurred vision, double vision, etc.
- High fetal heart rate, over 160 beats per minute
- Fatigue, exhaustion

Two key symptoms should be taken particularly seriously: rapid pulse and unexplained weight loss are not typical in pregnancy, and likely point to an overactive thyroid.

### Diagnosis

One of the main challenges for your practitioner is determining whether you are hyperthyroid due to GTT or Graves' disease.

Doctors cannot use the usual diagnostic tests—radioactive iodine uptake test or nuclear scanning—to diagnose hyperthyroidism during pregnancy because of the potential harm these tests pose to the fetus. Typically, ultrasound and blood tests for thyroid function and antibodies, as well as clinical evaluation of symptoms, will be used to make the diagnosis.

Initial testing usually includes TSH and free T4 tests. It's important to note that free T4 is essential, as the hormonal state of pregnancy makes total T4 less accurate. Antibody status is also frequently checked, to determine if your thyroid problem is due to Graves' disease, which is most often the case in pregnant women who are hyperthyroid.

Note, however, that in a normal pregnancy without any thyroid dysfunction, the pregnancy hormone HCG causes a small, temporary increase in free T4 levels toward the end of the first trimester; this may result in a reduction of TSH level to near-hyperthyroid levels. During this stage, one in five women actually have TSH levels in the hyperthyroid range, yet are not clinically hyperthyroid. A low-normal or borderline hyperthyroid TSH level in pregnancy should not automatically lead to a diagnosis of hyperthyroidism, as the thyroid will often return to the normal range during the second and third trimesters.

### Treatment

Radioactive iodine treatment (RAI) is never given to pregnant patients, because of the risk of destroying the baby's thyroid gland with radioactive material. This leaves antithyroid drugs and surgery as the treatment options for women during pregnancy.

Pregnant patients with hyperthyroidism should be monitored monthly. Pulse should be monitored, along with weight gain, thyroid size, TSH, and free T4 on a monthly basis. Fetal growth and pulse should also be monitored monthly. Ideally, pulse should remain below 100 beats per minute. Weight gain should be normal for pregnancy.

### Drug Treatment

All of the antithyroid drugs—PTU, methimazole, and carbimazole—have been compared in pregnancy. PTU and methimazole are category D drugs—known to be potentially harmful to an unborn baby. Babies of mothers taking antithyroid drugs have a higher risk of goiter, hypothyroidism, or even cretinism. The risk of hyperthyroidism to you and your baby are, however, greater than the risk of taking a low dose of the medication, so antithyroid drugs are used in pregnancy. Typically, your doctor will recommend the smallest possible dose that will control your condition. The goal is to keep the TSH level in the normal range, or borderline hyperthyroid, using the lowest possible dose of antithyroid drug. Some doctors have noted that since a somewhat increased heart rate is normal in pregnancy, it is not necessarily symptomatic evidence for antithyroid drug dosage to be increased.

The antithyroid drug methimazole (Tapazole) more easily crosses the placental membranes, meaning that there is a slightly greater risk to an unborn baby of side effects. In addition, rare instances of a condition called aplasia cutis, which causes scalp defects, have been seen in babies born to mothers who took methimazole during pregnancy. These scalp defects have not been seen in babies of mothers who took PTU. PTU is the most water-soluble of the drugs, and therefore doesn't transfer from mother to baby or into breast milk as efficiently as the other drugs. PTU is therefore the recommended drug during pregnancy. Outside the United States, there are some areas where PTU is not available; methimazole and carbimazole are regularly used during pregnancy, and no particular problems have been associated with careful use of these drugs.

All antithyroid drugs do cross the placenta, however, and excessive doses may produce goiter and hypothyroidism in your unborn baby. The objective, therefore, is to give you the smallest dose possible that will keep your free T4 in the upper end of the normal range and prevent dangerous hyperthyroidism symptoms. Your doctor will work to make sure that you are getting only that amount of drug that you need to control your hyperthyroidism.

The recommended daily dose of PTU in pregnancy is typically 200 mg or less, but no more than 300 mg. PTU levels under 150 mg a day are rarely associated with fetal hypothyroidism. (*Note:* If 400 mg or more is needed to control symptoms, your doctor may recommend a subtotal thyroidectomy during your second trimester.) For methimazole, the maximum daily dose is 20 mg.

*An Important Note:* Block/Replace antithyroid treatment—which combines antithyroid drugs with thyroid hormone replacement as a way to control hyperthyroidism—is not used during pregnancy, because the antithyroid drug will cross over the placenta to the baby, and can make the baby hypothyroid.

To accurately assess your thyroid levels, especially free T4, your doctor should perform thyroid tests every two weeks at the beginning of your treatment and every two to four weeks when your thyroid levels are normal.

Many of the most serious symptoms improve or go away entirely as the pregnancy proceeds, so your levels should be evaluated in the monthly tests. You may need to cut your antithyroid drug dosage—or even stop taking the drug entirely—

later in the pregnancy. Most doctors will not discontinue your antithyroid drug treatment until after week 32 of the pregnancy, because before that time the risk of relapse is high.

You should also be tested again in the early weeks after delivery, because hyperthyroidism will sometimes worsen in the postpartum period.

Beta-blockers may help with significant heart-related symptoms. You cannot, however, safely take them for more than a short period of time. Longer-term use during pregnancy is associated with various dangers to the fetus. Typically, doctors recommend that you use a beta-blocker for no more than two weeks, and they are most often given during the time when you are waiting for antithyroid drugs to take effect.

Iodide drugs should also not be given during pregnancy because they cross the placenta and may cause goiter and/or hypothyroidism in your baby.

### Surgery

In some cases, your doctor may recommend that you have your thyroid surgically removed in part, or in full, during pregnancy. If it's recommended, it's typically performed in your second trimester (when the greatest risk of miscarriage has passed, and before the third trimester, where there's a risk of preterm labor and delivery). Surgery may be recommended in the following cases:

- You are allergic to the antithyroid drugs.
- You have bad side effects from antithyroid drugs.
- You don't want to take the antithyroid drugs.
- You need extremely high doses of antithyroid drugs to manage your condition (more than 300 mg of PTU or more than 20 mg of methimozole a day).

- You are not responding to the antithyroid drugs, and still have significant symptoms.
- The fetus is showing evidence of hypothyroidism due to the antithyroid drugs (typically, a slow fetal heart rate or slowed bone development).

Second-trimester thyroid surgery is considered safe. You will, however, possibly need to start thyroid hormone replacement drugs at some point, so be sure that your thyroid levels are monitored regularly after surgery.

## Implications for Your Newborn

You may have concerns about the future health of your baby. Luckily, less than 2 percent of babies born to mothers with Graves' disease and hyperthyroidism are born hyperthyroid. That's more than a 98 percent chance that your baby will be completely free of thyroid problems.

Still, though, it bears mentioning that even if your hyperthyroidism is properly treated, your baby can experience problems.

Antibodies, called stimulating TSH receptor antibodies, or thyroid-stimulating immunoglobulins (TSI), can cross the placenta, causing an overactive thyroid in the fetus, known as fetal thyrotoxicosis. Fetal monitoring during pregnancy is therefore essential. Fetal thyrotoxicosis is suggested when the fetal heart rate is faster than 160 bpm. An ultrasound examination may reveal intrauterine growth retardation, fetal goiter, and advanced bone age as well. TSI levels should also be measured in the third trimester in all patients with Graves' disease. A high TSI level is more likely to be associated with fetal thyrotoxicosis.

Babies born to hyperthyroid mothers also need to have a blood test after birth to test for neonatal thyrotoxicosis. Approximately 1 percent of these infants will have the condition, which can cause stunted growth, irregular heart rate, bone problems, skull abnormalities, and other problems. If left untreated, the mortality rate can be as high as 30 percent.

Remember that you must advise everyone of your condition. While your doctor and your endocrinologist know that you're hyperthyroid, the attending physicians, pediatricians, and nurses at the hospital may not. Or the information may get lost or forgotten in the excitement and hullabaloo of childbirth and a new baby. So, with rare but possible scenarios such as neonatal thyrotoxicosis or newborn hyperthyroidism, it's absolutely essential that you let every health care provider who comes in contact with you know of your condition. If you feel that you may be unable to, appoint a patient advocate—your spouse, a friend, or another health care professional—to act on your behalf.

Also, your newborn may test completely normal at birth for any signs of hyperthyroidism, and be sent home with a clean bill of health. However, 7 to 10 days later, he or she may come down with hyperthyroid symptoms. Why? The PTU—or other antithyroid drug you took—may have passed through the placenta and bloodstream to your baby, hiding his or her hyperthyroid condition, which only becomes evident after the medications wear off.

Be on the lookout for potential symptoms of hyperthyroidism in your newborn.

- Excessive appetite with poor weight gain
- Normal appetite but poor weight gain
- Fast heartbeat

- High blood pressure
- Nervousness
- Irritability
- Bulging eyes
- Vomiting
- Diarrhea
- Difficulty breathing due to enlarged thyroid gland (goiter) pressing on windpipe

If you suspect hyperthyroidism in your infant, have the baby evaluated immediately by your pediatrician.

### A Note About Transient Hyperthyroidism of Hyperemesis Gravidarum

Some women who have severe morning sickness develop hyperthyroidism. This short-term hyperthyroidism, known as transient hyperthyroidism of *hyperemesis gravidarum*, or THHG, is accompanied by nausea and vomiting, along with typical hyperthyroidism symptoms such as rapid heart rate and anxiety. Weight loss is usually noticeable, especially since it occurs during pregnancy. Because of dehydration, you may need to be hospitalized to receive intravenous fluids. Treatment for THHG during the first trimester usually consists of a short course of antithyroid drugs. Pregnancy hormones normalize after the first trimester, and by weeks 16 to 20, many women will find that the hyperthyroid symptoms have subsided. TSH may remain suppressed, however, even while the thyroid function returns to normal. Treatment may then be able to be discontinued, and thyroid function usually returns to normal before delivery.

## Goiter

Goiter, or an enlarged thyroid, is fairly common in pregnancy. Ultrasound may be done to evaluate the thyroid enlargement. Typically, a fast-growing goiter may be treated with thyroid hormone replacement drugs. A slow-growing goiter that is not causing symptoms will most likely be treated with observation and monitoring during pregnancy. If the goiter is in a particularly dangerous location and makes breathing or swallowing difficult, surgery may be recommended.

## Thyroid Nodules in Pregnancy

Several studies have indicated that pregnancy can trigger the development of thyroid nodules, make existing nodules larger, and predispose the mother to developing a multinodular goiter later in life. Fortunately, in most cases, nodules don't pose a significant risk to your baby or you. Unless they are very large or ill placed (such as near the windpipe, where it can interfere with breathing), treatment can wait until after you've had your baby.

A 2002 study published in the *Journal of Clinical Endocrinology and Metabolism* examined the pregnancies of 221 women in their first trimester of pregnancy: 34 (15.3 percent) had thyroid nodules; of these, 12 (5.4 percent) had more than one nodule. Typically, the nodules enlarged during the pregnancy, in some cases to almost double their initial size, and remained enlarged as long as three months after delivery. New nodules appeared in 25 (11.3 percent) of the women as their pregnancies progressed, leaving the total incidence of thyroid nodular disease at 24.4 percent by three months after delivery. In this particular study, no malignancies were detected among the women in the study.

If nodules are detected during the first half of pregnancy (the first 20 weeks), a fine-needle aspiration biopsy will often be done to examine the cells of the nodule for cancer. A biopsy is definitely called for if the nodule is larger than 1 cm, is enlarging during pregnancy, or if there are palpable cervical lymph nodes.

If nodules are identified during the second half of pregnancy, some physicians will postpone the fine-needle aspiration biopsy until after delivery unless there is strong suspicion of malignancy. Many physicians will attempt to prevent growth of the nodule by giving you thyroid hormone replacement drugs. If growth is not stopped, then fine-needle aspiration biopsy is usually performed.

If the biopsy is highly suggestive of malignancy, thyroid surgery should be performed. If the biopsy is only mildly suspicious, then surgery is usually postponed until after delivery.

## Thyroid Cancer in Pregnancy

Thyroid cancer is still fairly rare, though it is on the increase. There were approximately 25,700 new cases of thyroid cancer in the United States in 2005. Of these, more than 19,000 were in women.

In general, the chance of a thyroid nodule being cancerous is about 5 percent; however, the risk is much higher in pregnant women. At a meeting of the American Association of Clinical Endocrinologists, researchers reported that in one series of studies, pregnant patients with thyroid nodules had a thyroid cancer rate of approximately 27 percent. The researchers speculated that pregnancy may promote thyroid nodule formation in general or speed up the growth of previously cancerous nodules.

Traditional methods of testing for cancer, such as a nuclear scan, are too much of a risk to the baby during pregnancy, so fine-needle aspiration is the optimal diagnostic method.

If thyroid cancer is diagnosed, the first decision is whether to remove the thyroid gland during pregnancy or wait until after the baby is delivered. Surgery during pregnancy may be advisable if a thyroid cancer is large, appears to be a more aggressive type of cancer, or has already spread to other sites in the neck or the body. When surgery during pregnancy is needed, doctors typically wait until the second trimester. Scheduling surgery during this period reduces the chance of interfering with the baby's early development or causing premature labor.

Surgery may also be delayed until after delivery if the thyroid cancer is small and there is no evidence that the cancer is aggressive or has spread. Delayed surgery may also be best if there are other risks to the pregnancy that may make surgery more risky. Several smaller studies have shown that delaying surgery does not increase the risk of spread, recurrence, or death in pregnant women with papillary thyroid cancer.

With or without surgery, treatment with thyroid hormone replacement drugs is started, in order to deactivate thyroid tissue until surgery can be performed. Free T4 and TSH lab tests should be done every one to two months to ensure that the medication is just high enough to suppress TSH.

After delivery and surgery, a decision must be made about whether to give radioactive iodine treatment. Radioactive iodine must not be given during pregnancy, as it can damage the fetus's thyroid gland. Similarly, radioactive iodine cannot be given until the mother has stopped nursing her baby.

Thyroid cancer treatment generally has a very high success rate; this applies to thyroid cancers discovered in pregnancy as well. A 1999 study reviewed the outcome of thyroid cancer found in nine pregnant women. One patient underwent a thyroidectomy in the middle of her pregnancy, while the others had the surgery 3 to 10 months postpartum. Seven of the malignancies were the papillary kind, and two were follicular, and measured anywhere from as small as 1 cm to as large as 6 cm. The patients were followed an average of 14 years, and all but one had an excellent prognosis.

## Who Should Monitor Your Thyroid During Pregnancy?

This is a good question. Endocrinologists will often tell you that your obstetrician should be following your care; and the obstetrician may refer you back to the endocrinologist or may not be able to monitor your thyroid proficiently or knowledgeably. Generally, you should consider having an endocrinologist oversee the thyroid aspect of your care while you are pregnant, because many obstetricians are simply not well versed in the latest thyroid treatment approaches.

One survey looked at obstetricians' level of knowledge about thyroid disorders, and typical treatment practices. While younger practitioners were more likely to identify and treat pregnant women for thyroid conditions, some 20 percent of the ob-gyns surveyed said that they don't regularly screen women for thyroid disorders. Only half of the ob-gyns felt that they had received adequate training in thyroid disorders during pregnancy. Few, unfortunately, felt that it was comprehensive. While more than 80 percent of the ob-gyns were confident that they could diagnose thyroid disease in a pregnant woman, fewer were confident in their ability to treat it.

Obstetricians and gynecologists also seem to routinely underestimate the implications of thyroid disease on pregnancy. Even the official ob-gyn practice guidelines for thyroid disease in pregnancy, last updated in 2002, claim that there is consensus and expert opinion that:

- Slight goiter during pregnancy does not warrant thyroid testing in a pregnant women if she doesn't have thyroid "symptoms."
- Women who have morning sickness do not need thyroid function tests.

The guidelines do not consider routine screening of pregnant women for thyroid disease. This is in opposition to recommendations from the National Institute of Child Health and Human Development (NICID), which has recommended that *all* pregnant women receive a routine TSH screening.

These issues point to the importance of having an endocrinologist as part of your health care team with experience managing thyroid disease in pregnancy.

# Chapter 8

# Infertility and Miscarriage

Surviving meant being born over and over.

—Erica Jong

P rimary infertility is defined as the inability to become pregnant after a year of trying to conceive if you are under 35, and after six months if you are over 35. Secondary infertility is inability to become pregnant after having had a successful pregnancy.

Age is an important factor, because it has such a bearing on fertility. Typically, in any given month, a woman in her twenties with an entirely normal reproductive system having unprotected sex has about a 25 percent chance of conceiving; after three months of trying, 60 percent will conceive without medical assistance. By the time a woman is 40, that rate drops significantly, and the likelihood of getting pregnant in any given month is approximately 5 percent.

Infertility is not uniformly considered a medical condition, and only some states require that medical insurance policies cover some level of infertility treatment.

Approximately 44 percent of women with infertility do seek medical assistance, however, and the vast majority—95 percent of women—who receive fertility treatment are treated with drug therapy or surgery; the remainder use advanced reproductive technologies such as in vitro fertilization (IVF).

## Infertility Causes and Risks

Fertility in women requires that various physiological processes function.

- The woman must have a supply of viable eggs.
- The woman must ovulate and release one or more viable eggs.
- The hormonal environment—estrogen, progesterone, etc.—must be generally capable of supporting ovulation, fertilization, implantation, and pregnancy.
- The ovaries, fallopian tubes, and uterus must not pose any structural or anatomical impediments to pregnancy.
- The cervical mucus has to be conducive to the sperms' movement and friendly to the sperms' survival.
- The uterine lining—the endometrium—must develop properly and be able to support a fertilized egg.
- The luteal phase—the time from ovulation to menstruation—must be long enough to allow for proper implantation and hormone production that will prevent menstruation—in the presence of a fertilized egg.

- There must be sufficient progesterone during the luteal phase and early weeks of the pregnancy to allow for proper development of the fetus.

There are a number of risk factors for infertility.

- Age: A woman's age is the key determining factor for fertility. Our fertility is optimal in our twenties. The probability of having a baby decreases by 3 to 5 percent each year after the age of 30, and at a faster rate after 40. Nowadays, however, more women than ever are delaying childbearing into their thirties and forties. Currently, as many as 20 percent of women have their first child after the age of 35. As women get older, the miscarriage rate also rises. In our early twenties, there's a 12 to 15 percent chance of miscarriage in each pregnancy, but in our 40s, the risk rises to 50 percent.
- Heredity: If our mothers or sisters have had problems conceiving due to various hormonal conditions or reproductive disease, we are more likely to face similar hereditary problems.
- Endometriosis: Endometriosis can result in cysts, lesions, adhesions, and scar tissue that make it more difficult to conceive.
- Polycystic ovary syndrome: This condition can cause irregular periods, no menstrual periods, lack of ovulation, and a variety of hormonal abnormalities that result in infertility.
- Infections and sexually transmitted diseases: Infections and STDs, such as pelvic inflammatory disease, chlamydia, gonorrhea, syphilis, herpes, and the human

papillomavirus (HPV), when not treated can cause a number of problems, such as scarred fallopian tubes, cervical changes, and other issues that may make it more difficult to get pregnant.

- Premature ovarian decline: A diagnosis of premature ovarian decline reduces fertility, due to the hormonal changes inherent to the condition.
- Premature ovarian failure: Premature ovarian failure implies severe and sometimes irreversible infertility.
- Smoking: Smoking does particular damage to fertility, because it affects the ovaries and causes rapid depletion of viable eggs. Smoking also increases the risk of miscarriage. Smokers typically go through menopause two years earlier than nonsmokers.
- Surgery of reproductive organs: Loss of an ovary, tubal ligation, or surgery for cervical dysplasia can make it more difficult to get pregnant. Let you doctor know if you have had such surgery. You may need medical intervention to conceive.
- Cancer: Cancer treatments, including radiation and chemotherapy, can damage the ovaries and cause fertility problems or infertility.
- Body weight: Being overweight by more than 15 percent or underweight by 15 percent can impair fertility.
- Overexercising: Competitive athletes or anorexic girls who compulsively exercise can suffer from infertility.

## Your Thyroid and Fertility

In addition to the various factors identified above, undiagnosed or insufficiently treated thyroid problems are to blame for infertility or impaired fertility in some women. The AACE estimates, conservatively, that at least 6 out of every 100 miscarriages are directly associated with thyroid hormone deficiencies during pregnancy. One important study found that serum TSH levels and thyroid peroxidase antibodies were higher among women with infertility compared with controls.

Unfortunately, doctors don't often consider an undiagnosed thyroid problem, and go on to far more in-depth and costly testing and even invasive fertility procedures before evaluating the thyroid.

Houston-based women's health and hormone expert Dr. Steven Hotze believes that thyroid should be the first course of action.

> When you're dealing with infertility, the first thing that should be suspected is hypothyroidism. Physicians should check a woman's thyroid status if she's having a problem with infertility and miscarriage. Before embarking on a million-dollar workup, I think that women with infertility should get a clinical trial of a small therapeutic dose of Armour Thyroid. How hard is that, how complicated is that?

Reproductive endocrinologist and fertility expert Andy Silverman, M.D., Ph.D., agrees, saying in an online interview at the Fertile Heart website:

> I learned very quickly that often patients come in who have subtle thyroid problems and if I don't do the blood tests, it might be months or years before they'll actually become symptomatic. Of course, there's a cost associated with these tests, but I find that if we do a thorough history and all the appropriate testing we can pick up the problem before

there's clinical evidence of it, and we can start treating a patient and avoid unnecessary procedures.

Unfortunately, many women have experienced recurrent miscarriages, been diagnosed as infertile, or encouraged to have expensive and invasive fertility treatments without even being tested for an underlying thyroid condition.

You can't assume that infertility workups will include thyroid tests. Despite thyroid disease being not only common, but a known cause of infertility and miscarriage, some practitioners surprisingly still do not conduct even basic thyroid tests, much less a more comprehensive thyroid panel, as part of a basic or in-depth fertility assessment. Patient advocate Marie Savard, MD, shares this story:

> A woman came to me with years of infertility for a simple checkup. She said she had tons of blood work from the infertility and didn't need to be tested. I insisted on a TSH because I felt her thyroid was a little enlarged. Her TSH was very high, in the 80s or more, and ultimately she got treated … and had 5 healthy kids of her own without fertility drugs. Her problem, after years of expensive and invasive infertility treatment, was a simple thyroid problem. Everyone pointed the finger at someone else, assuming the other person had checked the thyroid.

### Thyroid Imbalance Testing

Ideally, if you experience any fertility problems, you should have a comprehensive thyroid workup to rule out or identify any thyroid conditions. The tests should include TSH, total T4, and free T4 and T3. If thyroid test results are normal, but symptoms are suggestive of a thyroid condition, the TRH stimulation test is also highly recommended. You may have to argue for a TRH test, because it's not as well known or widely used, but it may be essential as part of a fertility evaluation. One study looked at women ages 25 to 34 experiencing infertility for more than two years due to anovulation or luteal phase problems. The women received TRH tests. They concluded that a TRH stimulation test in such patients should be mandatory. "Subclinical hypothyroidism may be of greater clinical importance in infertile women with menstrual disorders—especially when the luteal phase is inadequate—than is usually thought."

## Thyroid Autoimmunity Testing

While some practitioners recommend systematic screening of all infertile women for thyroid dysfunction, including thyroid autoimmunity, many doctors feel these antibody tests are unnecessary, because they aren't aware of the research linking thyroid antibodies to miscarriage. However, there is a strong argument for testing.

Among women with normal thyroid function, and no history of pregnancy loss, those who tested positive for thyroid antibodies during the first trimester of pregnancy had a 17 percent miscarriage rate—a level that is twice the 8 percent rate of women without thyroid antibodies.

In some women, the antibodies actually become elevated long before any thyroid symptoms appear, or before they affect the thyroid enough to cause functional changes that are seen in standard blood tests. So there are millions of women with evidence of autoimmune thyroid disease—a factor that can interfere with fertility and pregnancy—who don't even know it.

Some experts theorize that thyroid autoimmunity is evidence of some underlying immune dysfunction that may make you more likely to reject a developing fetus. Another theory is that even if thyroid levels are supposedly normal, the autoimmunity still causes subtle thyroid deficiencies or makes you less able to meet the thyroid-related demands of pregnancy.

There are numerous studies indicating a relationship between thyroid irregularities, including antithyroid antibodies, infertility, and recurrent miscarriages. According to scientists from the Foundation for Blood Research in Scarborough, Maine, miscarriages could be reduced if doctors included a thyroid screen and antibody profile as part of the regular battery of prenatal tests. In an article in the journal *Obstetrics and Gynecology*, researchers found that the presence of antithyroid antibodies increases the risk of miscarriage. One study found that as many as 31 percent of women experiencing recurrent miscarriages were positive for various thyroid antibodies. And a study detailed in the *Journal of Clinical Endocrinology and Metabolism* found that risk of miscarriage can be twice as high for women who have antithyroid antibodies.

Researchers have shown that antithyroid antibodies can also make in vitro fertilization less successful. According to fertility expert Dr. Gregory Sher,

The presence of antithyroid antibodies is associated with a variety of manifestations of poor reproductive performance. These range from infertility, through early miscarriage to prematurity, intrauterine growth retardation, other serious complications of late pregnancy, and even fetal death.

A number of studies have shown fertility improvements in women given thyroid treatment. Thyroid treatment can also improve the effectiveness of fertility treatments. For example, in one study of women who had thyroid antibodies, border-line hypothyroidism according to TSH levels, and a history of recurrent and early miscarriages, thyroid hormone was given before and during pregnancy. This significantly reduced the miscarriage rate, and 81 percent of the women had live births, versus only 55 percent of the women who were given intrave-nous immunoglobulin injections.

This is why tests for thyroid antibodies are particularly important when there are fertility issues. The relevant tests include thyroid peroxidase (TPO) antibodies test, thyroglobulin-antithyroglobulin antibodies test, and thyroid-stimulating immunoglobulin (TSI) test.

It is important to note that traditional blood tests for thy-roid antibodies do not identify one out of every five women with positive results. For a woman with recurrent pregnancy loss, then, more sensitive thyroid antibodies tests—known as enzyme-linked immunosorbant assays (ELISAs) or gel aggluti-nation tests—are required.

## Infertility Evaluations

While thyroid treatment may be a simple breakthrough solu-tion for infertility, it's also important to have a basic infertility workup.

Generally, the recommendation for women is that under 30, try for a year, and if you can't get pregnant, have a basic infertility evaluation. Women over 30 should try for six months, and then get evaluated. Women over 35 and women of any age who have irregular cycles may want to have a basic infertility evaluation right away. The recommendations are summarized in Table 3.

## TABLE 3. RECOMMENDATIONS FOR INFERTILITY EVALUATION

|  | REGULAR MENSTRUAL CYCLES | | IRREGULAR MENSTRUAL CYCLES |
| --- | --- | --- | --- |
|  | UNDER 35 | OVER 35 | ANY AGE |
| Women without thyroid disease | Try for a year before a basic infertility workup | Try for six months before a basic infertility workup | Have a basic infertility workup right away |
| Women with thyroid disease | Try for six months before a basic infertility workup | Have a basic infertility workup right away | Have a basic infertility workup right away |

A basic infertility evaluation includes:

- Medical history
- Physical examination
- Ovarian hormone assessment: determination that the ovaries can produce viable eggs. This is done by measuring the follicle-stimulating hormone (FSH) level on day 3 to determine the ovarian reserve. Luteinizing hormone (LH) is also measured to establish a baseline and determine if levels are sufficient to trigger the release of an egg.
- Blood work: In addition to the FSH and LH levels, key laboratory work done as part of a basic infertility evaluation may include assessment of reproductive hormones, including estradiol, progesterone, prolactin DHEA-S, testosterone, and thyroid
- Fallopian tube assessment: A basic infertility evaluation should also determine that your fallopian tubes are open and functional. To establish this, you will usually need

to have a procedure known as a hysterosalpingogram (HSG). In an HSG, a dye is injected into the uterus. An X-ray is taken to look at the shape of the uterus, make sure that the fallopian tubes are not scarred, and identify any fibroids, polyps, tumors, or structural problems that may interfere with pregnancy.

- Semen analysis: A basic infertility examination should also include a semen analysis for the man to determine that he is producing normal sperm and seminal fluid.

*Note:* Some practitioners include a basic TSH test, or a more thorough thyroid panel (TSH, free T4, free T3) as part of their basic infertility evaluation, but surprisingly, *many do not routinely test for thyroid disease in infertile patients.* You cannot assume that thyroid evaluation is part of your blood work: you may have to ask for it specifically. In fact, you should insist on a complete thyroid panel as part of your basic blood work.

If you haven't been tested, your doctor may also run tests to determine if you have immunity to rubella (German measles) and varicella (chicken pox), because these two common diseases are particularly dangerous to pregnant women, and immunizations might be recommended before you try to become pregnant.

Typically, a follow-up to the first visit of a basic infertility evaluation will occur on the day of your LH surge before ovulation, so that LH levels can be measured and evaluated to see if they are sufficient.

## In-Depth Testing

A woman is considered to be experiencing recurrent pregnancy loss (RPL) after two consecutive miscarriages. After two miscarriages, the risk of another miscarriage goes up to from 26 to 40 percent, and more in-depth testing is in order.

## Ultrasound Tests

Ultrasound tests may be useful to evaluate a number of factors, including the thickness of the uterine lining, the status of follicles, and the uterine and ovarian anatomy and condition. In some cases, ultrasounds are done several days apart, to monitor the development of follicles and release of an egg. Ultrasounds can be abdominal—the transducer is passed over the abdomen—or transvaginal—the transducer is a long, slender probe that is inserted vaginally.

## Hysteroscopy

If anything questionable is seen on the HSG, your doctor may want to take a more in-depth view, which typically requires a procedure called a hysteroscopy. Hysteroscopy involves inserting a small scope or camera through the cervix, into the uterus, to examine abnormalities up close. The procedure, done under local or general anesthesia, is able to also get pictures. Carbon dioxide gas may be used to expand the uterus and allow for a better view.

## Laparoscopy

In laparoscopy, again a small scope is inserted, but this procedure is done under general anesthesia. The scope is inserted through a small surgical incision in the naval, and carbon dioxide gas is used to expand the abdominal cavity for examination of the uterus, fallopian tubes, and the ovaries. A second incision, usually in the pubic hairline, is made to insert an instrument for manipulation.

## Endometrial Biopsy

If the uterine lining appears at all abnormal, an endometrial biopsy is done. This is usually done in conjunction with a hysteroscopy, right before the onset of menstruation, and tissue from the endometrium is scraped to evaluate the lining thickness.

## Cervical Mucous Tests

This postcoital test evaluates whether sperm can penetrate and survive in the woman's cervical mucous. It includes a bacterial screening of the mucous.

## Testing for Infection

Since infections and diseases can impair fertility, testing may be done for the following conditions:

- Ureaplasma
- Mycoplasma
- Gonorrhea
- Chlamydia
- Syphilis
- Toxoplasmosis
- Cytomegalovirus (CMV)
- Hepatitis B and C
- HIV

## Chromosomal Testing

A small percentage of fertility problems are due to chromosomal irregularities or defects, and chromosomal testing can help identify these problems. Chromosomal testing can be done on fetal miscarriage tissue, but only if the tissue can be obtained at the time of a miscarriage or during a dilatation and curettage. Karyotyping of parents is chromosome analysis of the blood of both parents. It can show if there is a potential problem with one of the parents that leads to miscarriage, but it often has to be done in conjunction with fetal testing to provide answers. These tests help rule out the approximately 3 percent of parents who carry a "hidden" chromosomal problem—called a balanced translocation.

## Immunologic Testing

Some experts estimate that as much as 40 percent of unexplained infertility—and 80 percent of unexplained miscarriages—may be due to immunologic problems. For a woman who has a history of autoimmune disease, or who had more than two miscarriages, especially if she's over 35, immunologic testing may be helpful. Immunologic testing is also recommended for women who produce viable embryos through in vitro fertilization procedures, but embryos fail to implant.

Immune dysfunction isn't always easy to target. For example, a woman may appear to be unable to become pregnant, when in reality, she is getting pregnant but not sustaining the pregnancy in the earliest days. Hormones don't prevent a menstrual period, and the embryo is lost. In that situation, the immune system is causing rejection of the embryo in the first few days after fertilization. Often, such a pregnancy is undetectable.

The immune system can also attack the fertilized and newly implanted embryo as a foreign body, causing a first-trimester miscarriage.

If you have Hashimoto's thyroiditis or Graves' disease, are receiving what your doctor feels is optimal treatment for your thyroid condition, and have plotted your menstrual cycles and fertile periods and attempted conception for a year (if you're under 30), or six months (if you're over 30), you may want to consider moving forward with immunologic testing to determine if you have any factors that may prevent successful pregnancy.

Immunologic testing is also recommended for women with the following indications or risk factors:

- Two miscarriages after the age of 35
- Two IVF or GIFT failures after age 35
- Three miscarriages before age 35
- Three IVF or GIFT failures before age 35
- Poor egg production (fewer than six eggs) upon stimulation with fertility drugs
- One blighted ovum: a placenta develops, but there is no fetus visible on ultrasound at no later than around six weeks in the pregnancy
- Previous autoimmune or immune test results, e.g., tested positive for antinuclear antibodies or rheumatoid factor
- Diagnosis of rheumatoid arthritis, lupus, multiple sclerosis, or other autoimmune diseases
- Previous pregnancies where the baby had intrauterine growth retardation
- One living child and more than one miscarriage while attempting to have a second child

### Inhibin B Test

Day 3 inhibin B levels are considered more accurate and direct in assessing ovarian reserve than a traditional FSH test. The results of this test can also predict the response of ovaries to fertility drugs.

### Antinuclear Antibodies Test

Antinuclear antibodies (ANA) measure the immune system's inappropriate response to various components of cells.

They are seen in a number of autoimmune and immunologic diseases, including lupus, Sjögren's syndrome, scleroderma, and many other diseases. Many of these conditions can interfere with proper placental development and cause early miscarriage. Some studies show that positive ANAs are seen in as many as 22 percent of women with recurrent miscarriage and nearly half of all women who have infertility and failed attempts at IVF.

### Anti-Ovarian Antibodies Test

The anti-ovarian antibody test identifies the body's inappropriate immune response to the ovaries, which can cause failure to ovulate, irregular ovulation, poor implantation, and failure of various fertility treatments. Anti-ovarian antibodies are found in some 70 percent of women with premature ovarian failure. AOA are also more common in women with thyroid disease, Addison's disease, and endometriosis.

### Anti-Sperm Antibodies Test

The anti-sperm antibodies test evaluates the existence and level of female antibodies that target components in sperm. An estimated 10 percent of women with fertility problems have antibodies to sperm, which can prevent conception.

### Anti-Phospholipid Antibodies Test

A common autoimmune factor that affects pregnancy is the existence of anti-phospholipid antibodies, or APA. These antibodies are proteins that circulate in the bloodstream. They can interfere with coagulation, prevent blood from flowing properly, and cause clots that compromise the blood flow to the reproductive organs, cut off oxygen and nutrition to the uterus and placenta, and generally prevent implantation and pregnancy or cause miscarriage. If a woman tests positive for various APA, it shows that there is an underlying autoimmune problem that is likely to prevent the phosopholipids from operating properly, which puts the woman at risk for miscarriage, second-trimester pregnancy loss, and many other dangers to pregnancy.

APAs develop after a woman has had several miscarriages, IVF failures, endometriosis, or tissue injury in the reproductive area. Autoimmune diseases, including Hashimoto's and Graves' disease, can also cause a woman to make APAs. As many as 22 percent of women with recurrent pregnancy losses are thought to have APAs, and the more pregnancy losses a woman has, the higher the level of these antibodies.

There are a number of different types of APAs, but the most important tests focus on identifying

- Anti-phospholipid antibodies (APA)
- Anti-cardiolipin antibodies (ACA)
- Lupus anticoagulant (LAC)

Without detection or treatment, the live birth rate among women with APAs ranges from about 10 to 20 percent, but with treatment, it's thought that women with APAs have a live birth rate of 70 to 80 percent.

### Thrombophilia Panel

Thrombophilia is defined as a predisposition for thrombosis, or blood clots. A variety of problems in pregnancy have been linked to various forms of thrombophilia. A thrombophilia panel may include a number of tests:

- Antithrombin
- Activated partial thromboplastin time (APTT)
- Factor V Leiden coagulation
- Homocysteine
- PAI-1
- Protein C
- Protein S
- Prothrombin

### Immunoglobulin Panel

Many autoimmune disease patients have abnormal immuno-globulin tests, and these are also common in women who have recurrent miscarriages and infertility. Evaluation of immuno-globulins should be done before possible treatment with intra-venous immunoglobulin (IVIg) is considered.

### Embryo Toxic Factor

The embryo toxic factor (ETF) test evaluates the potential for an immunologic reaction to fetal tissue, which causes first-trimester miscarriage.

### Natural Killer Activity

Natural killer cell activity measures the cytotoxic capability (ability to kill cells) in each cell. Women with increased NK levels have higher rates of implantation failure and miscarriage, because these NK cells are also found in the uterine tissue. Some patients with high NK cell activity respond very well to IVIg therapy to suppress the immune response earlier in the pregnancy and avoid rejection of the fetus. Live birth rates can go from 20 percent among untreated women to as high as 80 percent among some treated groups.

## Surgery to Treat Infertility

Some conditions such as cysts, scar tissue, adhesions, and fibroids warrant surgery to correct anatomical or structural impediments to pregnancy. Some of the surgeries that are done to address underlying conditions, thereby restoring or enhancing fertility, include:

- Tubal anastomosis (reversal of tubal ligation or sterilization)
- Fallopian tube reconstruction
- Surgery for endometriosis
- Surgical removal of uterine fibroids
- Surgery for adhesions and scar tissue
- Reconstructive surgery of birth defects involving the uterus and vagina
- Surgical treatment of ovarian cysts
- Repair or removal of hydrosalpinx-damaged fallopian tube
- Removal of uterine fibroids
- Surgical removal of endometrial polyps
- Tubal cannulation to unblock fallopian tubes

## Infertility and Assisted Reproduction Drugs

There are no treatments that are considered capable of "turning back the clock" on a woman's ovaries. There are, however, treatments that can make the best of the ovarian function that remains, improve fertility, and increase the chance of pregnancy. These treatments can

- Increase the number of eggs that develop
- Enhance the chance that the egg might be fertilized
- Provide supplemental hormones, such as progesterone, that are required to sustain a fertilized egg
- Help avoid an immune reaction that attacks the semen, the ovaries, or the embryo itself

### Antibiotics

Various antibiotics are prescribed for both partners when infectious diseases such as ureaplasma, chlamydia, or micoplasma are identified. While the role of infection in infertility is still a fairly unexplored area, some practitioners believe that treating these underlying infections may help restore fertility in some women.

### Clomiphene Citrate

The drug clomiphene citrate, commonly known by its brand names Clomid and Serophene, helps fertility by supporting the pituitary in stimulating development of follicles. Clomiphene is given for five days, starting on days 3 to 5 of the cycle. Research has shown that among women given clomiphene, as many as 80 percent will ovulate normally.

Clomiphene essentially tricks the body into responding as if there is no estrogen, and the pituitary gland secretes more luteinizing hormone and follicle-stimulating hormone. Around 10 percent of the time, clomiphene causes more than one egg to develop, so there is a higher frequency of multiple pregnancies in women taking this medication. While clomiphene stimulates the follicle development, it doesn't ensure ovulation. Some women also require an injection of HCG to trigger ovulation.

Clomiphene can actually impair fertility in women who are ovulating regularly, so it should be used only in women who have specific ovulation problems. Some newer studies have theorized that longer-term use of clomiphene (more than 12 cycles) may increase the risk of ovarian cancer.

### Superovulation Drugs

There are a number of drugs designed to help fertility by stimulating ovarian follicle growth. These medications are used for women with polycystic ovary syndrome (PCOs), and as part of intrauterine insemination (IUI) or in vitro fertilization procedures These drugs are typically given on days 2 or 3 of the cycle, for from 6 to 9 consecutive days. The ovaries are monitored by ultrasound and blood tests to watch for "superovulation"—the production of multiple eggs. (The pregnancy success of these drugs is mainly due to the production of a number of eggs.) When follicles reach a particular size, and there are sufficient estrogen levels, HCG is injected to trigger ovulation, which then occurs 36 to 48 hours later.

Three medications include only follicle-stimulating hormone (FSH). Bravelle is a urinary-derived FSH, but it is rarely prescribed. The most prescribed FSH drugs, however, are synthetic, recombinant FSH: Gonal-F and Follistim. These drugs are identical in structure to human FSH, but are derived from recombinant DNA technology. About 95 percent of the FSH drugs used in the United States for infertility fall into this category. They are considered purer, more consistent, and more effective than human-derived FSH.

There are also three popular menotropin drugs, also known as human urinary-derived gonadotropins, or HMG. These are injectable drugs that include both FSH and LH and have been available for more than three decades. Menopausal women excrete very high amounts of FSH and LH in urine, and the menotropin drugs are made by obtaining and purifying the urine of postmenopausal women and extracting the FSH and LH. The three main drugs in this category are Pergonal, Repronex, and Humegon.

These drugs run a risk of multiple pregnancies, and up to 50 percent of pregnancies using these drugs result in multiple births, most often twins. There are some concerns about a potential link between these drugs and an increased risk of ovarian cancer, but the link has not been definitively established.

### Human Chorionic Gonadotropin

When follicles are ready and ovulation needs to occur, human chorionic gonadotropin (hCG) can be injected to trigger ovulation; hCG is used before IUI or IVF. It is available in generic form or as Pregnyl and Novarel (human, urinary-derived hCG preparations) and Ovidrel (recombinant hCG). Like the recombinant FSH, the hCG is considered purer, more consistent, and more effective than human-derived hCG.

### GnRH Analogs

Premature ovulation or LH surge can prevent successful pregnancy when using superovulatory drugs. For this reason, some doctors prescribe drugs known as GnRH analogs, which stop FSH and LH production. There are two types of medicines in this category:

- Gonadotropin-releasing hormone (GnRH) agonists, including Lupron and Synarel. These drugs stimulate full release of FSH and LH, and eventually this turns off the FSH and LH release
- GnRH antagonists, including Cetrotide and Antagon. These drugs turn off FSH and LH within several hours of one injection.

## Bromocriptine and Cabergoline

The drugs bromocriptine (Parlodel) and cabergoline (Dostinex) are orally administered drugs that reduce the pituitary gland's production of prolactin and combat hyperprolactinemia. Women who are experiencing infertility due to ovulation problems that result from hyperprolactinemia may benefit from these drugs. Pills are taken daily, but discontinued in pregnancy. The drug is considered safe to use, even for several years. It's estimated that as many as 50 percent of women with hyperprolactinemia will ovulate and be able to become pregnant as long as they follow this treatment.

## Progesterone

Progesterone is essential in pregnancy because it not only helps prepare the lining of the uterus for implantation of a pregnancy, but if pregnancy occurs, it helps maintain the pregnancy. If there is insufficient progesterone, a pregnancy has very little chance of success.

Progesterone is used in many ways to help enhance fertility and support successful pregnancy:

- During fertility treatments with superovulatory drugs for intrauterine insemination or in vitro fertilization—usually after ovulation or egg retrieval
- During early pregnancy (through the first trimester) to supplement low progesterone levels

For fertility and pregnancy support, prescription progesterone should be used. These are micronized progesterone preparations that are almost identical to human progesterone. These can include:

- Progesterone in oil (PIO) by injection: This is considered the best form of progesterone supplementation for patients having fertility treatments, as it can deliver a high level of progesterone very quickly.
- Prometrium: This is oral progesterone in capsule form, which needs to be taken several times a day to maintain proper levels.
- Progesterone vaginal suppositories: These are custom-compounded by pharmacists, and as they melt in the vagina, they release progesterone into the uterus. Because the progesterone has a local effect, blood tests cannot be used to monitor the effectiveness.
- Crinone or Prochieve: This is a progesterone vaginal gel that comes in prefilled applicators. These are generally less messy than suppositories. Again, because the progesterone has a local effect, blood tests cannot be used to monitor the effectiveness.

## Treatment for Immunologic Causes of Recurrent Pregnancy Loss

Treatment for immunologic causes of fertility and pregnancy problems vary, based on the cause.

## Anticoagulants: Aspirin and Heparin

Anticoagulants are primarily used for women who have anti-phospholipid antibodies. The theory behind use of anticoagulants is that they help prevent blood clots from forming in the vessels to the placenta, and improve blood flow to the uterus. Anticoagulants can also help improve implantation rates in women with a thin uterine lining.

Aspirin functions as a prostaglandin inhibitor, and low-dose adult aspirin therapy (81 mg) is sometimes recommended for women who have implantation failures and pregnancy losses after implantation. Aspirin therapy is also given to some women having in vitro fertilization procedures.

Several studies of women with anti-phospholipid antibodies who had experienced recurrent pregnancy loss show that the women receiving aspirin had a live birth rate of 44 percent. The success rate jumped to 80 percent in women receiving aspirin plus the anticoagulant drug heparin, which is given by injection.

## Intravenous Immunoglobulin

Intravenous immunoglobulin IVIg—is produced from human-derived antibodies. Donor blood is pooled, washed, processed, and made into the IVIg, which helps to prevent immune-triggered rejection of the fetus.

IVIg works by:

- "Blocking antibodies"—providing antibodies to antibodies
- Suppressing the body's production of autoantibodies
- Enhancing regulatory immune cell activity
- Suppressing natural killer cell activity

Maximum effectiveness is seen with IVIg treatment that starts prior to conception and continues through the sixth month of pregnancy. IVIg can be very expensive: treatment for a single pregnancy can run as high as $10,000.

In one study, women who had two or more miscarriages with no identifiable cause received either IVIg or placebo treatment. In the study of 95 women, 47 received IVIg and 48 received placebo. After four cycles, 61 women were pregnant, resulting in 29 live births and 32 miscarriages. Among the women who delivered a baby during the study, 18 were from the IVIg group, compared to 11 from the placebo group, showing that IVIg could enhance the chance of live birth. Another study showed live birth rates of 62 percent among women who had recurrent miscarriages receiving IVIg, compared to 33 percent among women receiving placebo.

### Steroids: Prednisone, Prednisolone, and Dexamethasone

Steroid therapy using prednisone, prednisolone, or dexamethasone can both prevent preimplantation pregnancy failure and postimplantation pregnancy loss in women with immune dysfunction. Many in vitro fertilization protocols include steroid drugs. They are started before drugs are given to stimulate ovulation and continue until pregnancy is established. Prednisone is sometimes used with aspirin for anti-phospholipid antibody treatment, but studies have shown that the heparin-aspirin combination is equally or more effective and has fewer side effects than the prednisone treatment. Prednisone can reduce antibody levels, and so it may be helpful in early pregnancy for antithyroid antibodies, as well as other autoimmune antibodies, to help prevent rejection of the fetus.

## Phosphodiesterase Inhibitors

Phosphodiesterase inhibitors are drugs that have an anti-inflammatory effect and can help increase blood flow. Drugs in this category include sildenfil (Viagra) and pentoxiphylline (Trental). Both can increase blood flow to the uterus. In one study, women who used Viagra in vaginal suppository form had increased uterine blood flow and lining thickness; 42 percent of the women also had successful pregnancy, after recurrent IVF failure.

## Lymphocyte Immunotherapy

One recent study found that women having lymphocyte immunotherapy or lymphocyte immune transfusion (LIT)—also known as white blood cell immunization—who have had several previous lost pregnancies or attempts at embryo transfer have better results with LIT prior to the transfer.

## Intralipid

Intralipid is a fat emulsion that when given intravenously may help enhance the success of implantation and sustain pregnancy. Intralipid is comparatively inexpensive, and since it's not a blood product, it poses fewer risks of contamination and may have some benefits for infertility patients.

## Plasmapheresis

Plasmapheresis is a procedure where, like dialysis, the blood is filtered. In this case, antibodies are filtered out of the blood, and the patient is infused with immunoglobulin, which includes regular antibodies for healthy immune function.

## Assisted-Reproduction Techniques

Assisted-reproduction techniques can help achieve pregnancy for some women. Some of the popular techniques used to help achieve pregnancy are described here.

### Intrauterine Insemination

Intrauterine insemination (IUI) can help fertility by increasing the number of sperm available to fertilize the egg. Since only 1 of 2,000 sperm ejaculated into the vagina actually make it to the fallopian tube, direct insemination can help improve the odds. IUI is also used with superovulation drugs. According to some experts, after three cycles, IUI has on average a conception rate of around 36 percent.

### Gamete Intrafallopian Transfer

In gamete intrafallopian transfer, known as GIFT, superovulatory drugs are used; eggs are produced and then mixed with sperm in a dish. The eggs and sperm are then transferred back to the fallopian tubes so that the fertilization can occur in the body, and the embryo can then develop naturally from that point.

### Zygote Intrafallopian Transfer

Zygote intrafallopian transfer, known as ZIFT, is similar to GIFT, except that instead of the sperm-and-egg mixture, an actual fertilized egg—the zygote—is returned to the fallopian tubes. The embryo can then develop naturally from that point.

### *In Vitro Fertilization*

In vitro fertilization, known as IVF, is a technique whereby, after a superovulatory cycle, the best eggs can be selected and mixed with sperm in a culture dish in a laboratory. In some cases, additional techniques such as intracytoplasmic sperm injection (ICSI)—where sperm are directly injected into the egg—is used to achieve fertilization.

The success rate of IVF varies depending on the clinic, the woman's characteristics, and approaches used, but age is a factor. Many fertility clinics won't accept women over age 44 for treatment unless they are willing to use a donor egg from a younger woman. Generally, the live birth rate for each IVF cycle started is age-related:

- 30 to 35 percent live births for women under 35
- 25 percent live births for women ages 35 to 37
- 15 to 20 percent live births for women ages 38 to 40
- 6 to 10 percent live births for women over 40

### *Donor Egg or Donor Embryo*

If you are unable to use your own eggs for conception, a donor egg can be fertilized and implanted in your uterus, or a donor embryo may be implanted.

## Natural or Holistic Fertility Approaches

Entire books have been written just about holistic or alternative medicine approaches to fertility. I can touch upon only some high points here.

Toni Weschler's book *Taking Charge of Your Fertility: The Definitive Guide to Natural Birth Control, Pregnancy Achievement, and Re-*

*productive Health* is required reading. You will also want Nicky Wesson's *Enhancing Fertility Naturally: Holistic Therapies for a Successful Pregnancy* and Helen Caton's *The Fertility Plan: A Holistic Program to Conceiving a Healthy Baby* to round out your holistic fertility library.

## Food and Nutrition

Having a healthy diet is important to help support fertility. This means a diet as free of processed foods as possible, avoiding foods like white flour and sugar, staying away from hormones in meat and dairy, and using organic produce whenever possible. You'll want to make sure your diet has enough low-fat protein in it—without enough protein, estrogen is less available, and fertility can be compromised. A variety of nutrient-rich fruits and vegetables, good whole grains, and seeds and nuts rich in vitamins are all important.

Many fertility experts suggest that you avoid alcohol, artificial sweeteners like aspartame, and even your home's tap water, unless it has been safety tested. You can check with the EPA for information on the safety of your home water supply.

Some practitioners suggest that you avoid coffee and caffeinated soft drinks, but some studies have found that drinking tea, including caffeinated tea, can actually improve fertility.

Months before conception, you'll definitely want to start a supplement that includes 400 mcg of folic acid at least 30 days before fertilization, along with a prenatal vitamin that includes iodine.

A good multivitamin rich in antioxidants, and a high-potency vitamin B complex can also be helpful.

## Herbal Medicine

There is a long tradition of herbal medicine for fertility enhancement. If you are interested in herbal fertility help, you'll want to consult with an herbal medicine expert with expertise in fertility treatment for specific guidelines and formulations unique to your own situation. Here are a few key points to keep in mind.

- Chasteberry is thought to reduce prolactin levels, and increase LH levels and progesterone.
- L-arginine, an amino acid, is also recommended to help with circulation to the uterus.
- Helonias-viburnum is considered a uterine tonic that is good for women with a history of miscarriage.
- Red clover blossoms and leaves have some blood-thinning properties and are also thought to help make cervical mucus more favorable to a longer survival of sperm.
- Nettle leaf is thought to thicken the endometrium and improve the environment for implantation of a fertilized egg.
- Raspberry leaf is a commonly used tonic for reproductive health.
- Dong quai (tang kwei) root is a popular Chinese herb used as a female tonic and to help utilize estrogen properly. It should not be taken in pregnancy, as it may stimulate contractions.

## Traditional Chinese Medicine

Traditional Chinese Medicine (TCM) typically includes a combination of both acupuncture and herbal treatments to help resolve imbalances and restore health. Because Traditional Chinese Medicine is customized for the individual, you would need to see a trained, reputable practitioner of this ancient art and science. TCM can help to regulate the menstrual cycle and hormones, balance the endocrine system, strengthen the overall constitution, and prepare the body to support a pregnancy. TCM can also be used to help support overall health and make assisted reproductive technologies more effective.

It is not a quick-fix approach, however. It can take several months of treatment to achieve some balance in a younger woman, and women closer to 40, who smoke, and those who have had more extensive fertility treatment, such as fertility drugs, hormonal supplements, assisted reproductive technologies, or who have hormonal conditions, all require from six months to a year before seeing some results.

Dr. Randine Lewis, who incorporates TCM into her practice, says in her book *The Infertility Cure* that with patients who follow a TCM treatment program faithfully over time, she has a pregnancy success rate of approximately 75 percent.

### Lifestyle Changes

There are some basic lifestyle changes you'll want to incorporate for enhanced fertility.

- Stop smoking. Smoking impairs fertility, increases the risk of miscarriage, and if you do get pregnant, it's harmful to an unborn baby, not to mention your own health. Avoid secondhand smoke exposure as well.
- Avoid recreational drugs. These include marijuana, cocaine and ecstasy. Eliminate recreational use of prescription pain medications, tranquilizers, and other drugs as well.

- Minimize or avoid exposure to the chemicals found in household cleaners.

## Weight and Exercise

Weight and exercise are both important issues for fertility. You want to normalize your weight as much as possible, for maximum fertility. Being overweight, especially by more than 15 percent, can impair fertility, just as being underweight, especially by more than 15 percent, can also hurt fertility.

Excessive exercise—such as training for a marathon, being a professional athlete or a gymnast, etc.—may cause amenorrhea or change hormone levels so as to make pregnancy very difficult to achieve. While you want to exercise for general health, flexibility, aerobic health, and muscle strength, avoid overexercising.

## Mind-Body Approaches

Many experts point to the role of stress in fertility. If you are functioning in a state of stress or anxiety, not only does this have a serious hormonal impact discussed throughout this book, but it simply does not allow your body to function optimally. This can affect fertility and reproductive capabilities.

Some alternative practitioners recommend mind-body therapies for stress reduction and relaxation to help enhance fertility. Overall, mind-body techniques and the relaxation response have as their objective calming the mind, achieving a peaceful state, coping with stress, relaxing the body and mind, generating a "relaxation response," expressing and clearing emotions, changing negative thoughts, and controlling physical functions such as breathing.

There are many mind-body therapies to choose from, and you'll need to explore those that appeal most to you. Some of the suggested approaches include the following:

- Psychotherapy, counseling
- Biofeedback
- Guided imagery
- Hypnosis
- Yoga
- Tai chi
- Meditation
- Prayer or spiritual healing
- Creative therapies: music therapy, art therapy, dance therapy
- Breathing exercises
- Support groups
- Reiki or energywork

# Chapter 9

# Postpartum and Breastfeeding Challenges

> If pregnancy were a book they would cut out the last two chapters.
>
> —Nora Ephron

The period following childbirth can be difficult for any new mother, regardless of whether or not you have thyroid difficulties. For some, there's pain—especially if you've had a difficult or prolonged labor, or a Cesarean section—sleep deprivation, worry, and the emotional upheaval of adding a baby to your household. Fluctuating hormones, signaling the end of pregnancy and triggering the start of lactation, can trigger dramatic mood swings. And we've all heard about the "baby blues," a period of time when you may feel unexplainably sad or depressed.

But it's not as commonly known that the postpartum period can trigger a variety of thyroid and hormonal problems, even among women who have never had any thyroid problems prior to pregnancy. In fact, according to the America Association of Clinical Endocrinologists, as many as 18 percent of women are diagnosed with postpartum thyroiditis.

## The Postpartum Period for Thyroid Patients

If you are already hypothyroid when you have your baby, be sure to have your thyroid levels tested in the week after delivery. Dosage changes are often needed, and keeping your thyroid on track can help you successfully adjust during the postpartum period. Pay close attention to symptoms of any hormonal imbalances, and have all your hormone levels tested periodically, including thyroid, progesterone, testosterone, and estrogen levels.

Pregnancy and the postpartum period can be a rollicking roller-coaster ride of hormones, and an imbalance can have serious consequences, such as severe depression. Let's take a look at typical hormones at work in pregnancy, and how they "crash and burn" after childbirth.

Progesterone, also dubbed the pregnancy hormone, is roughly 300 times higher than normal, in order to sustain the growth of your baby. Estrogen also rises significantly, with estradiol 100 times higher than normal, and estriol about 1,000 times the nonpregnant level. Because of the higher hormonal level, most pregnant women report feeling happy and healthy.

Shortly after delivery, however, hormone levels come crashing down, throwing the new mother into an emotional upheaval.

Some doctors recommend natural progesterone to treat postpartum depression. Still others, noting the tendency of depressed people to have lower quantities of serotonin in their brain chemistry, prescribe medications to raise the level of the hormone responsible for calmness and a general sense of well-being.

Whatever your doctor prescribes, just make sure that there are no other contraindications with any other medications you are taking.

In my case, when my daughter was around 5 months old, I still couldn't shake the exhaustion and a moody feeling that had descended on me about a month after her birth. I went to my regular doctor, sure that I must be suffering from postpartum depression. The doctor, however, decided to run some hormone tests before recommending an antidepressant. It's a good thing she did, because she discovered that I had various hormonal imbalances in addition to my thyroid edging out of normal range into hypothyroid TSH levels again. She prescribed some natural progesterone and changed my thyroid hormone dosage. Very soon, it was as if the fog had lifted and the world was a happy place again.

## Postpartum Hair Loss

Women typically experience a good deal of hair loss after delivery, regardless of whether they have a thyroid condition. During pregnancy, you may have happily noticed that your hair seemed thicker and fuller. That's because pregnancy hormones generally lessen hair loss. Postpartum, however, those hormones drop drastically, and the hair starts falling out. Generally hair loss take place for about four to six months after childbirth. But for women with postpartum thyroid issues, hair loss can be quite severe and long-lasting, in some cases. Massive clumps can fall out in the drain or shower, and the hair itself can change texture, becoming coarse, brittle, or easily tangled.

The good news is that if you are getting treatment for your thyroid condition, what seems like a startling amount of hair loss will gradually slow down, and then cease, once your hormones are in the normal range. This may take longer than you like, but rest assured, I've had many thousands of e-mails from people, and have yet to hear from anyone who lost all his or her hair, or became bald, due to thyroid disease. But people have experienced significant loss of hair volume. In my case, I lost almost half my hair. I had long, thick hair, and it got much thinner at various times, in particular, the time after delivery. My hair got so thin that if I gathered all of it together to make a ponytail, it was as thick as a pencil! You can bet that got my attention. Luckily, because of some of the approaches I describe in the following section, my hair did eventually return to normal.

Generally, most people with hypothyroidism lose hair all around the head, rather than in patches. Here are a few tips for dealing with hair loss, beyond getting treated for your thyroid dysfunction. *Note*: With any supplements or prescription drugs, check with your physician before starting them if you are breastfeeding.

*Make sure it's not your thyroid drug.* If you are hypothyroid and taking Synthroid as your thyroid hormone replacement, and you are still losing hair, you may need to switch brands or drugs. Prolonged or excessive hair loss is a side effect of Synthroid for some people. Many doctors do not know this, even though it is a stated side effect in the Synthroid patient literature.

*Make sure you're not undertreated.* Hair loss can also result from being undertreated—not being at the right TSH or not taking the right drugs for you. So if your TSH is below 0.5 or above 2, it may be contributing to hair loss.

*Find out if you need a second drug.* I am also one of the people who does better and has less hair loss on a T4-T3 drug versus pure synthetic T4 only (like Synthroid). Over the years, I've taken both Thyrolar and Armour Thyroid, and both have worked far better for me than Synthroid.

*Consider supplements*. When I have had major bouts of hair loss (despite low-normal TSH and being on a T4-T3 drug), I took the advice of Dr. Stephen Langer. In his book, *Solved: The Riddle of Illness,* Langer points to the fact that symptoms of essential fatty acid insufficiency are very similar to hypothyroidism; he recommends evening primrose oil, an excellent source of essential fatty acids, for people with hypothyroidism. The usefulness of evening primrose oil, particularly in dealing with the issues of excess hair loss with hypothyroidism, was also reinforced by endocrinologist Kenneth Blanchard, author of *What Your Doctor May Not Tell You About Hypothyroidism.* According to Dr. Blanchard,

> For hair loss, I routinely recommend multiple vitamins, and especially evening primrose oil. If there's any sex pattern to it—if a woman is losing hair in partly a male pattern—then, the problem is there is excessive conversion of testosterone to dihydrotestosterone at the level of the hair follicle. Evening primrose oil is an inhibitor of that conversion. So almost anybody with hair loss probably will benefit from evening primrose oil.

As someone who has had a few periods of extensive hair loss since I became hypothyroid, I can vouch for the fact that taking EPO was the only thing that calmed it down. It not only slowed, then stopped my hair loss over about two months, but new hair grew back, and my hair was no longer strawlike, dry, and easily knotted. When I take EPO, I usually take 500 mg, twice a day.

*Consult a doctor for a prescription treatment.* After delivery and completion of breastfeeding, you can also consult with a dermatologist to work with you on drug treatments, including scalp injections, drugs like Rogaine (minoxidil) and Propecia, and other treatments that may help with hair loss.

## Postpartum Thyroiditis

Many doctors don't think of the thyroid when evaluating troublesome symptoms in a new mother. New mothers who go to the doctor with complaints of fatigue, depression, anxiety, heart palpitations, and irritability may condescendingly be told these are normal for new mothers, "go home and try to rest and relax, and enjoy your baby." Worse yet, the doctor may write a prescription for a medication, such as an antidepressant, that the woman does not need, instead of testing her and treating an undiagnosed thyroid problem.

During pregnancy, the body's immune system is suppressed—a process known as immunosuppression—in order to protect the baby. Normally, the immune system would seek out and "attack" something it perceives as foreign, like a fetus, but the immunologic changes during pregnancy protect the baby from immune system attacks. After childbirth, however, the body's seek-out-and-attack abilities can return, but they can malfunction, and turn on its own organs, glands, tissues, and cells.

For some women, the immune system decides that the thyroid is the target of attack, and the woman develops postpartum thyroiditis: her body starts manufacturing antibodies against the thyroid. The antibodies either cause too much thyroid hormone to be released into the bloodstream (making her hyperthyroid) or damage the thyroid tissue and make it less able to produce hormone (making her hypothyroid).

Postpartum thyroiditis was only recognized as a distinct condition in the 1970s. It's essentially a transient, short-term thyroiditis that occurs in the postpartum period, typically during the first year after birth.

Postpartum thyroiditis is common, and is thought to occur in anywhere from 5 to 9 perent of women after pregnancy. Women with type 1 diabetes have three times the risk of postpartum thyroiditis, compared to nondiabetic women. PPT is also more common in a woman who has had a previous episode.

Women who test positive for antithyroid antibodies early in their pregnancies have a 33 to 50 percent chance of developing thyroiditis after childbirth. However, postpartum thyroid problems also can appear in women who tested negative for the antibodies, so this suggests there are other risk factors for developing postpartum thyroid problems.

- A personal or family history of thyroid disease
- A goiter
- Type 1 diabetes
- History of postpartum thyroiditis in prior pregnancies

### Symptoms

Typically, a woman with postpartum thyroiditis enters the hyperthyroid phase first, followed by the hypothyroid phase; she may then bounce between the two—several times, even—before things settle down.

Often, the hyperthyroid episode starts at around 14 weeks postpartum, and the hypothyroidism is seen around 19 weeks postpartum. (Less commonly, a woman can move right to the hypothyroid state.) In general, however, the condition begins with hyperthyroid symptoms, including:

- Feeling particularly warm or hot, especially when others are cold
- Weak muscles, especially arms and legs
- Feeling anxious, nervous, or irritable
- Hand tremors
- Rapid heart rate, fast pulse
- Generally weak or fatigued feeling
- Weight loss
- Diarrhea
- Exhaustion
- Insomnia
- Hair loss
- Low milk supply when breastfeeding

All of these symptoms can be easily mistaken for symptoms some women experience after pregnancy, making it harder for doctors—and patients—to recognize the underlying condition.

Marisol describes her postpartum symptoms:

> I was feeling depressed, had pain in my hands and feet, swelling, weight gain, hair loss, candida, anxiety, very low energy; I couldn't function without caffeine or sugar...the list goes on.

The hyperthyroidism symptoms typically shift into hypothyroidism symptoms:

- Extreme fatigue and exhaustion
- Constipation

- Problems with memory and concentration
- Feeling cold when others are warm or hot
- Dry skin
- Muscle cramps, body aches and pains
- Weight gain
- Hair loss
- Low milk supply when breastfeeding

Frequently, the postpartum symptoms cycle back and forth between hypothyroidism and hyperthyroidism.

One important note: typically, pain and tenderness in the thyroid area is common in regular thyroiditis, but rare in postpartum thyroiditis.

Kiley, who had her first child at almost 39, started experiencing symptoms in the year after childbirth.

> I started to have trouble sleeping at night. I also started to feel depressed. My skin dried up like an old prune, my vagina was dry as could be, and I had zero sex drive. I suspected a hormonal imbalance of some kind, but assumed it was the sex hormones, since my sex drive was so absent. I worked long-distance with a holistic chiropractor who ran a battery of tests for me, one of which was thyroid antibodies. That test was the key to my recovery. I found out my antibodies were elevated—I had Hashimoto's.

Five months after she had her first baby, Lena's husband threatened to check her into the hospital to find out what was wrong with her.

> My TSH was in the 60s!! I was at a point where I could only speak words (not sentences) to my husband and my mother. I couldn't read, not even a street sign, couldn't think at all. It's

a wonder I was able to take care of the baby. I often lost my car in the parking lot, gained a bunch more weight despite dieting, and was extremely confused all the time.

Lena had another bout of postpartum thyroiditis after a subsequent pregnancy.

I lost my cell phone and wallet almost every day. I had episodes of what I call temporary amnesia. I would find myself driving on a highway with my kids sleeping in the back and wonder, Where am I? Where am I going? Where have I been? Or my son would be in preschool and I would not see him with me and panic—Where is he? Sometimes I would remember quickly; other times I would have to call someone and get directions home or be filled in on reality. My brain stabilized back to normal after six months.

### Diagnosis

As discussed in Chapter 3, blood tests will typically be done to help identify the nature of the thyroid problem postpartum. If true postpartum thyroiditis is suspected, in order to make an accurate diagnosis, your health care provider first needs to distinguish postpartum thyroiditis during the hyperthyroid period from Graves' disease. To diagnose Graves', he or she may want to perform a radioactive iodine uptake test. A diagnosis of Graves' disease would show a high reading of radioactive iodine uptake, while postpartum thyroiditis would show a low one.

If you are breastfeeding, you'll need to stop for three to five days, since radioactive iodine can appear in breast milk and permanently damage the baby's thyroid gland. Pump and store as much milk as possible to cover the time when you can't breastfeed; after the scan, "pump and dump" to keep your supply up (i.e., use a breast pump and discard the milk until you've been given the all-clear signal).

Hypothyroidism in the postpartum period is defined as a TSH level greater than 3.6 (lower than the 5.0 to 6.0 upper limit of the normal reference range) with an elevated free T4.

### Treatment

For some women, no treatment is necessary for postpartum thyroiditis, and the condition resolves on its own. A majority of women will return to normal several months to a year after postpartum thyroid diagnosis, and will never have another problem. Other women have postpartum thyroid problems after every pregnancy, but otherwise things return to normal until menopause, when thyroid problems again appear. Some women—possibly as many as 30 percent—remain hypothyroid because the thyroid gland was too heavily damaged by the imbalance or because the pregnancy activated an inherent case of autoimmune thyroid disease.

For those who are hypothyroid and are prescribed thyroid hormone replacement drugs, your thyroid should be periodically evaluated (TSH, free T4, free T3) and your dosage gradually tapered off as your thyroid levels return to normal.

For those who are temporarily hyperthyroid and require treatment, beta-blockers are typically given to relieve some of the symptoms of an overactive thyroid. More radical treatments like antithyroid drugs, surgery, or radioactive iodine treatment (RAI) are usually not done for postpartum thyroiditis manifesting with hyperthyroid levels and symptoms because it's not always known if the situation will be permanent.

Once you've had an episode of postpartum thyroid problems, you are more likely to develop a thyroid problem during a period of stress, subsequent pregnancy, or menopause.

## Postpartum Depression

Clearly one of the more crippling side effects of postpartum thyroiditis is depression. While it's true that many healthy women suffer from the blues shortly after childbirth, in most cases it lasts only a few weeks. With postpartum thyroiditis, the depression can stretch on for months if you don't seek help, and it tends to be far more severe. Antithyroid antibodies are linked to the development of postpartum thyroiditis, and some studies find that testing positive for antibodies early on in pregnancy raises the risk of postpartum depression.

Simply because you have postpartum thyroiditis, it doesn't sentence to you to months of depression. Some women have all the signs of thyroid problems after childbirth, but aren't depressed. A Spanish study, reprinted in a 2001 issue of the *Journal of Clinical Endocrinology*, studied 641 pregnant women and tested them for signs of both depression and postpartum thyroid problems at regular intervals following childbirth; 11 percent of them had some form of postpartum thyroid dysfunction, 7.8 percent had postpartum thyroiditis, and 1.5 percent of them were diagnosed with Graves' disease. Since only a small number were diagnosed with postpartum depression, the authors concluded that women with postpartum thyroid problems were not more likely to suffer depression. They did note that people with a history of depression were at risk of another bout of depression after childbirth.

Should you have depression, however, it's vital to keep track of your T3, T4, and TSH levels and follow your doctor's orders carefully. And if you are being told that your levels are "normal," but you still can't shake the depression, insist on being seen again, and ask your doctor if your medication can be adjusted. You may need a new dosage, a second drug, or a combination of two drugs. You may be undertreated: your doctor may feel that symptoms should disappear or greatly diminish with a TSH level of 3. You, however, may not feel well until your TSH is at 1 or 2. Good communication with your health care provider about your symptoms and general state of well-being is essential. The first year of your baby's life is far too important to spend in a fog of sadness and depression.

*Important:* If you are having any thoughts of hurting yourself or your baby, *get help immediately!* Call 911 or a suicide hotline, a minister, rabbi or priest, a child abuse prevention hotline, or your doctor. Take this very seriously! There is help for how you feel. You are not alone.

### Thyroid Disease That Begins Postpartum

For some women, postpartum thyroid problems are not temporary. Pregnancy is a trigger, and the thyroid imbalances that show up after the birth are the start of a lifelong autoimmune thyroid disease, such as Hashimoto's or Graves' disease. It is sometimes difficult to differentiate between a postpartum thyroid problem and a lifelong thyroid disease that appears postpartum.

Typically, in the hyperthyroid phase, the radioactive iodine uptake test can differentiate between postpartum thyroiditis and Graves' disease. Graves' disease is likely to be a more permanent condition, while the hyperthyroidism of postpartum thyroiditis almost always resolves, and the thyroid swings to a hypothyroid phase.

Differentiating postpartum hypothyroidism from a permanent thyroid condition may be harder, because it's estimated that as many as 20 to 30 percent of women who become hypothyroid after pregnancy will remain so and require lifelong treatment. Many doctors treat a postpartum hypothyroid women for one year, then have the woman stop taking thyroid hormone temporarily so levels can be retested.

Women with transient hypothyroidism after pregnancy who are treated and then stop treatment should still have a thyroid evaluation annually, as some experts have reported that as many as half of these women are again hypothyroid seven years after childbirth.

Generally, treatment for Hashimoto's disease and the hypo- or hyperthyroid conditions that result is the same in the postpartum period as at other times. In the case of Graves' disease, however, women cannot continue to breastfeed after receiving radioactive iodine (RAI) treatment, so they may choose to forgo RAI, and instead use antithyroid drugs, which can in some cases be used safely while breastfeeding.

## Thyroid-Related Breastfeeding Problems

No doubt you are well aware of the benefits of breastfeeding an infant. The American Association of Pediatrics says that "human milk is uniquely superior for infant feeding." Breastfed infants reportedly score better on IQ tests, are sick less often, and enjoy better overall health. Breastfeeding mothers lower their risk of breast cancer and other types of cancer and use up more calories; they may return to their prepregnancy weight sooner by nursing their infants. Only around 22 percent of mothers in the United States breastfeed, however. For some, breastfeeding isn't feasible, due to work schedules or other issues. And there are mothers who try to breastfeed but find it difficult, or nearly impossible.

There are a number of problems that women can face that make breastfeeding physically difficult—pain, inverted nipples, mastitis infections, or a baby that has a poor suck reflex. But one particular problem—low milk supply—is very common. Unfortunately, low milk supply is often the reason a woman gives up trying to breastfeed entirely.

## Low Milk Supply Problems

The hormone prolactin is responsible for the production of breast milk. It is stimulated by thyrotropin-releasing hormone (TRH) which in turn stimulates TSH. When your levels of TRH are low, as they are in hypothyroid women, prolactin is insufficient and you may have difficulty producing enough breast milk to nourish your baby. So it is not uncommon for hypothyroid women to have low milk supply. However, many doctors and breastfeeding experts do not make women aware of this potential problem.

Specific signs that your baby is getting enough milk include:

- Five to six soaking wet disposable diapers (seven to eight cloth diapers)
- Two to five yellow, runny bowel movements each day in the first month. (After that point, it's considered normal for the baby to have one bowel movement a day, or even just 4 to 5 a week.)
- Regular weight gain of about 3.5 ounces per week

If your newborn isn't gaining weight after the first week, and isn't having the requisite number of soiled and wet diapers each day, he or she might not be getting enough milk due to low milk supply.

A complete thyroid evaluation (TSH, free T4, and free T3 tests) is essential for anyone having milk supply problems. The earlier you have the thyroid evaluated, the more likely that treatment may restore supply and allow for normal breastfeeding.

## Breastfeeding with Hypothyroidism

If you are hypothyroid before pregnancy, or are diagnosed with hypothyroidism while breastfeeding, you may have a difficult time with milk supply. It's not a guarantee, but if it does happen, realize that you are by no means alone, and there are many things you can do. I've detailed a number of suggestions later in this chapter.

One of the most common concerns about breastfeeding with hypothyroidism is whether you should continue taking your thyroid hormone drugs when you're breastfeeding.

Thyroid hormone replacement, when provided in the proper dosage level, crosses into breast milk in only minute quantities and has no adverse effect on the baby. Stopping your thyroid hormone, or taking less than prescribed, is not recommended, because insufficient treatment puts you at risk for various symptoms and side effects of hypothyroidism. And getting proper thyroid hormone replacement is actually necessary for milk supply and normal breastfeeding.

That said, if too much thyroid hormone is being taken and levels become hyperthyroid, then thyroid hormone can pass into the breast milk. For this reason, you must take medication as prescribed by your physician. The period following delivery is one when thyroid levels can fluctuate, so frequent testing is very important. Your dosage and thyroid levels may be just right three months postpartum, but three months later, the same dosage could be making you hyperthyroid. So plan to get blood levels drawn frequently (at least every three months) as long as you are nursing your baby.

A mother may think that if her baby is diagnosed as hypothyroid, she can take the thyroid hormone herself and have it pass through the breast milk to the baby. This is not an effective way to treat hypothyroidism in an infant. If a baby is found to be hypothyroid (usually by the mandatory heel stick test conducted on all newborns in the United States), the baby will need thyroid treatment right away to normalize thyroid levels. Untreated hypothyroidism in newborns must be treated immediately; otherwise, the baby is at risk of growth delays and developmental impairment. The amounts of thyroid hormone that pass into breast milk are not sufficient to act as a substitute for direct treatment for hypothyroidism in a newborn.

## Breastfeeding with Graves' Disease and Hyperthyroidism

The period after having a new baby is a time when some women's symptoms of Graves' disease and hyperthyroidism first appear. If you develop symptoms of Graves' disease or hyperthyroidism postpartum, your doctor will need to evaluate your condition. If you are breastfeeding during this time, there are some particular considerations to keep in mind.

### Getting Diagnosed

Some practitioners like to do a thyroid scan as a way to diagnose Graves' disease or hyperthyroidism. This procedure, however, is not recommended for a breastfeeding mother. A thyroid scan involves an injection of radioactive iodine. The radioactive iodine will pass into the milk for weeks and can concentrate in the baby's thyroid, causing damage to the baby's thyroid gland. If a doctor suggests a thyroid scan, you can ask the doctor whether an alternative diagnostic procedure—for example, blood test or fine-needle aspiration—can be performed instead of the scan. Or you should ask the doctor if the test is necessary in the first place. The primary reason for a scan in a nursing mother is to determine whether you have postpartum thyroiditis (frequently, a temporary condition), not Graves' disease.

If a scan absolutely needs to be done, it is possible to use technetium, rather than radioactive iodine. According to Dr. Jack Newman, "Technetium has a half life [the length of time it takes for half of all the drug to leave the body] of 6 hours, which means that after 5 half lives it will be gone from the mother's body. Thus, 30 hours after injection all of it will be gone and the mother can nurse her baby without concern about his getting radiation." During the time that the technetium is leaving the body, the mother should "pump and dump"—pump milk and dispose of it.

There is also the issue of radioactive iodine (RAI) treatment. While RAI is the most popular treatment for Graves' disease and hyperthyroidism in the United States, it must be deferred in women who are breastfeeding. The radioactive iodine appears in the breast milk and can pose a danger to the infant's thyroid. If a woman's Graves' disease or hyperthyroidism cannot be controlled with antithyroid drugs, and she does not want to stop breastfeeding and have RAI treatment, then the other option is surgery.

## Antithyroid Drugs While Breastfeeding

In the past, women taking antithyroid drugs as a treatment for an overactive thyroid were told to avoid breastfeeding entirely. But doctors modified this position somewhat in recent years.

There have been concerns that the antithyroid drugs methimazole (Tapazole) and carbimazole (Neo-Mercazole) may cause thyroid suppression and goiter in nursing infants. Many doctors still advise that this drug not be used; if it is used the breastfeeding infant's thyroid function should be checked at least every three months while the mother is on antithyroid drugs. According to the RxList drug information database online, "Postpartum patients receiving Tapazole should not nurse their babies." The American Association of Pediatrics, however, has approved these drugs for nursing mothers, and they are rated as "moderately safe."

The antithyroid drug propylthiouracil (PTU) is less controversial. The American Association of Pediatrics has approved if for use during breastfeeding, and rated it in the "safer" category, making it preferable to Tapazole and Neo-Mercazole. In one controversial study, hyperthyroid mothers who were breastfeeding continued taking PTU after delivery despite elevated TSH levels (indicative of PTU-induced hypothyroidism) in their newborns. The TSH levels of the newborns normalized, even though the mothers continued on PTU therapy; this indicated that PTU treatment of breastfeeding mothers may be safe for their babies. Another study of nursing mothers taking 150 mg a day of PTU found no evidence of neonatal hypothyroidism in the first three weeks of life. Some experts say that for PTU, doses as high as 750 mg a day can be taken by a breastfeeding mother without ill effects on the thyroid status of the infant.

For any mother using antithyroid drugs, careful monitoring of the breastfeeding infant's thyroid function is needed, at least every three months while the mother is on antithyroid drugs.

Tapazole and Neo-Mercazole are usually taken once a day, but PTU can be divided throughout the day, so some doctors

suggest taking PTU in divided doses after each feeding to minimize exposure.

Despite studies showing the safety, some doctors are not
convinced that breastfeeding should be encouraged in women
taking antithyroid drugs. A July 2000 study in *Pediatrics* found
that more than one-third of pediatricians and endocrinologists still advise against breastfeeding for those mothers taking PTU. They cite concerns over potential nonthyroid side
effects, for example, autoimmune disorders such as lupus and
arthritis.

Generally, however, some endocrinologists would say that
Tapazole or Neo-Mercazole of less than 20 mg a day, and PTU
of less than 150 mg a day pose a low risk, and that mothers on
this level of drugs shouldn't be advised against breastfeeding.
Infants should, however, have their thyroid function monitored
regularly.

Other drugs sometimes prescribed for Graves' disease and
hyperthyroidism, including beta-blockers (such as Proprano-
lol/Inderal or atenolol) or calcium channel blockers are generally approved by the American Academy of Pediatrics for use
in breastfeeding mothers.

## Other Breastfeeding Aids

Assuming that you've gone back to the doctor and had a full
panel of hormone and thyroid tests done, and medications adjusted as needed, your next step is to get professional breastfeeding advice.

A certified lactation consultant can check the baby's latch
on to the nipple, give you ideas for different ways to hold your
nursing infant, and suggest a number of helpful ways to increase milk supply and get your baby sucking more vigorously
and efficiently—all of which can help with milk supply.

You can find a certified lactation consultant at your hospital, a birthing center, through a recommendation from your pediatrician, in the Yellow Pages, or from La Leche League. La Leche can provide advice and support in your efforts to successfully breastfeed. To find a local group, visit the website at http://www.lalecheleague.org/leaderinfo.html.

### Proper Latch, Emptying Breast

It's particularly important to your milk supply that your baby is latching-on correctly, sucking well, and emptying your breast during a feeding. To tell if the baby is positioned correctly, his or her lips should be on your areola (the darker skin area of the breast), behind the nipple. A lactation consultant or La Leche League leader can observe and quickly tell you if your baby is effectively latching on.

To encourage proper sucking, consider limiting or avoiding pacifiers and bottles entirely, and avoid use of nipple shields. If supplemental formula is necessary, you can feed with a dropper, cup, or supplemental nursing system, to avoid interfering with the baby's ability to suck.

You may want to apply a warm compress to your breasts before feeding or massage the breasts during feeding; both techniques help with the let-down reflex, and encourage milk production.

### Timing

The more you breastfeed, the more milk your body is stimulated to produce, so frequency of nursing helps maintain and increase milk supply.

You'll want to encourage your baby to breastfeed frequently and as often as he or she wants, at least every two to three hours. Never go longer than five to six hours. You may even want to wake your baby up for an extra nighttime feeding if you have a baby who will sleep more than four or five hours.

If you have a sleepy or low-key baby, offer the breast more often, to encourage frequent nursing.

Let your baby end the feeding, either by falling asleep or detaching from the breast, usually after at least 10 or more minutes of active sucking and swallowing.

### Switch Nursing and Double Feeding

Milk supply may also be maintained or increased by doing something called switch nursing, also called "burp and switch nursing." Breast milk contains a watery foremilk at the beginning of a feeding, designed to quench the baby's thirst. High-fat, creamy, satiating hindmilk is produced as the baby continues to suckle. Allow your baby to feed on the first breast until the suck lessens in intensity and the baby becomes sleepy, then burp, and start over on the other breast. When sucking slows, repeat the process, switching again so the baby nurses at least twice at each breast.

You can also try double feeding: nurse your baby until he or she is satisfied; keep the baby upright and awake; burp, and 10 to 20 minutes later, nurse again.

Double nursing and switch nursing both stimulate more milk production.

### Pumping

Even if you are breastfeeding, pumping milk can help increase milk supply, especially if the baby is not nursing effectively or frequently enough to help maintain supply.

You may want to pump your breasts for five minutes after a feeding to fully empty the breast and stimulate more milk production.

Some women have also found that pumping between nursing sessions can help increase supply.

If your baby is unable to properly latch on or suck, then pumping milk and giving it to the baby in a bottle, dropper, or supplemental nurser is also an option to make sure your baby gets breast milk.

## Nursing Vacations and Self-Care

Some experts recommend a "nursing vacation" for milk supply problems. Contrary to what you might think, a nursing vacation is not when you stop nursing and head to the Riviera. While tired, frazzled new mothers might certainly enjoy dreaming about such a prospect, the nursing vacation is a way to boost your milk supply, bond with your baby, and get him or her on the path to weight gain.

Basically, you and your baby take to your bed (or comfy chair, or whatever room you feel most relaxed in) and do nothing but nurse—on demand and on schedule, every two hours or so. Make sure you have an adequate supply of fluids—nursing mothers can get very thirsty, and a well-hydrated mom is likely to produce more milk than a dehydrated one. Shelve all your obligations for another time—no cleaning the house, answering e-mail, running errands. A day or two on a nursing vacation is sometimes what's needed to jump-start milk production.

Proper self-care is also essential. Take time to rest and relax during the day. Get enough sleep, if possible (not always easy with a new baby!). Try to get extra help from family members or friends if you need it.

An effective way to help stimulate milk production is to nap and nurse. If you take a nap while nursing your baby, it helps increase the milk-producing hormones; and the rest is good for your body.

### Contact

Skin-to-skin contact during breastfeeding can help both mother and baby. If you undress your baby down to a diaper, this can help wake him or her and stimulate feeding. This close contact and bonding with your baby also helps with milk production and encourages let-down of more milk.

### Don't Smoke

Not only does nicotine enter breast milk and get to your baby, but it can decrease your milk supply. (Breastfeeding advocates will tell you that if you do smoke, they still want you to breast-feed, though this is a somewhat controversial recommendation.)

### Diet and Liquids

While there is no one miracle food that will suddenly boost your milk supply, doctors and lactation experts agree that a well-balanced diet, one filled with good, healthy foods with plenty of protein, calcium, and iron will go a long way in supplying a lactating mother with the energy she needs.

Generally, a nursing mother needs to continue the healthy diet she followed during pregnancy. Most lactating mothers need an extra 500 calories a day. Now is not the time to go on a crash diet to get back into those prepregnancy jeans, particularly when your baby is not feeding and gaining weight well.

Keep in mind that the extra 500 calories does not give you carte blanche at the Krispy Kreme counter. A few extra glasses of milk, a yogurt, a whole-grain sandwich, or a fruit smoothie will do the trick.

Drink plenty of fluids—particularly water—to refresh and rehydrate you before, during, and after nursing, and to increase the chances of better milk production.

Aim for at least 8 to 12 glasses of water a day. Try to avoid caffeinated diet sodas; they tend to have a dehydrating effect, and the jury is out on the safety of artificial sweeteners, especially as they can be passed on to your baby via your breast milk.

## Galactagogues

There are numerous medicinal herbs out there that are supposed to be galactagogues—they help increase milk supply—and some may be effective for you. It's always a good idea to check with your health care professional before taking any herb or tincture. Similarly, it's vital that you inform him or her if you are taking these alternative therapies, so he or she can check for any possible reactions or contraindications to your thyroid treatment or any other condition you may have.

### Fenugreek

The most commonly recommended herb for increasing milk supply is fenugreek, a galactagogue that should be available at your local health food store, drugstore, or vitamin supply store. It can be bought either in capsule form or as a tea, which is not quite as potent as the capsules. The typical dose is two to three capsules (580–610 mg each), three times daily. Some women achieve results quite rapidly—often in as little as a day or two—while others report a longer waiting period. Still others report no effect. Fenugreek has a pleasant maple scent and taste, and some mothers may find that they have a mild maple aroma about them for a while. There are no clinical studies proving the effectiveness of the product, but many do report increased milk supply after taking the herb. Fenugreek can be used as long as necessary. *Note:* Fenugreek should not be used in pregnancy, as it is a uterine stimulant.

### Blessed Thistle

Some women report success after using this galactagogue. While there are no clinical trials, herbalists say thistle stimulates the blood flow to the breast, making it easier for milk to flow. The herb reportedly also has antidepressant qualities. It's used either in capsule form or as a tincture (which many say works better than capsules). As many as 20 drops, two to four times a day, is said to be the best dose for increasing milk production. There are some serious caveats to the use of blessed thistle, however. Anyone who is allergic to plants in the daisy family should probably not take this herb, as it could trigger an allergic reaction. In large doses, the plant can cause vomiting, so users should be careful not to overdose. Blessed thistle can also stimulate menstrual flow, so it should not be used during pregnancy.

### Alfalfa

Alfalfa is sometimes recommended as a galactagogue, either by itself or in combination with fenugreek and blessed thistle. Alfalfa is not recommended for anyone with an autoimmune thyroid disease. Persons with systemic lupus erythematosus should avoid alfalfa at all costs, as alfalfa can aggravate or exacerbate conditions of lupus, including causing kidney damage.

Because people with other autoimmune conditions, including thyroid disease, are at a slightly increased risk of developing lupus, it's safest to not take alfalfa at all. If you are drinking a tea purported to increase milk supply, check the label ingredients for alfalfa, and discard the tea if it's there.

### Prescription Medications

Galactagogue medications help increase milk supply, and some doctors will prescribe them, provided all other avenues to breastfeeding success have been exhausted. Metoclopramide (Reglan) is available in the United States and is sometimes used to increase milk production. If you get a prescription for it, the typical dose is 10 to 15 mg, three times a day. It's a temporary drug, to be used no longer than four weeks.

One important caveat: If you suffer from depression, as many thyroid patients do, particularly in the dicey postpartum period, this drug is probably not for you. Some of the side effects of Reglan include depression and mood swings.

If you live outside of the United States, you may be prescribed domperidone (Motilium) to increase milk supply. Because domperidone has fewer side effects and reportedly is more effective and can be used for a longer time period, some lactation consultants recommend it over Reglan.

## When You Need to Use Formula

Sometimes, in spite of your best plans, things don't work out with simple breastfeeding. After exhausting all possible ways to get your baby gaining directly at the breast, you may need to supplement nursing or pumped breast milk with bottles, cups, tubes, or syringes of formula while trying to get baby nursing and gaining better. There are nonherbal, nonmedicinal ways of trying to stimulate more milk to flow, and some of these might work for you.

## Supplemental Nursing System

The supplemental nursing system is a device designed to give the baby adequate nutrition (pumped breast milk or formula) through a tube worn on the mother's chest, while still allowing the infant to suckle at the breast, hopefully stimulating milk flow.

There are different designs, but typically the milk or formula is held in a pouch or bottle that rests on the mom's chest. A small tube runs from the pouch, is taped to the mother's breast, and then into the baby's mouth.

## Cup or Syringe Feeding

As you may imagine, the nipples on a baby bottle and the nipples on a mother's breast are quite different, and a certain type of suck is needed for each one. Sometimes, when a newborn is switched back and forth from breast to bottle to breast to bottle, it creates a syndrome called "nipple confusion." The baby may get so confused by the two that he or she may not feed well on either, or may develop a preference for the bottle nipple, which is somewhat faster and initially easier to learn.

To preserve nursing and prevent nipple confusion, lactation consultants often recommend feeding the infant with a tiny cup or syringe. Most of these are available through the hospital, lactation consultants, or online (Medela.com sells a variety of specialty feeding devices). The cups and feeding products feature marked measurements so you can keep track of how much fluid your baby drank.

Whatever happens, as long as you know in your heart that you gave breastfeeding the best effort that you could, don't feel guilty if it doesn't work. You are not a failure, nor does the fact that you are not nursing reflect poorly on your mothering skills or your love for your infant. You tried everything you could possibly do, you sought out help from professionals, you followed their advice to the letter. It didn't work out. No guilt allowed! So pat yourself on the back for giving your baby the best start in life he or she could get!

### Avoiding Soy Formula

If you need to use formula, how can you choose which one to use? If you have to or choose to use formula, some studies suggest that staying away from soy formulas for infants is a good idea, particularly if you have thyroid conditions in your family.

Why? According to environmental scientist Dr. Mike Fitzpatrick, infants fed a steady diet of soy formula are more at risk for developing thyroid disease. Soy baby milks—and other soy products, for children and adults alike, he attests—have high levels of isoflavones, which are strong antithyroid agents.

According to Dr. Fitzpatrick, the New Zealand Ministry of Health "has found that infants with a history of thyroid dysfunction should avoid soy formulas and soy milks. Additionally, there is potential for isoflavone exposure to cause chronic thyroid damage in all infants fed soy formulas." Fitzpatrick stated that exposing infants to isoflavones was unnecessary and that the risk of harm could be avoided if manufacturers removed isoflavones from soy formulas. "In the interim," he stated, "it is appropriate for medical practitioners to monitor the thyroid status of infants fed soy formulas."

In the 1950s and 1960s, there were several studies involving a higher increase in goiter among children fed soy formulas. Since then iodine has been added to most soy formulas, but the goitrogenic (goiter-producing) isoflavones are still present.

Experts estimate that thyroid dysfunction is on the rise, as is the rate of thyroid cancer. Some people—though certainly not all soy researchers—point to the increased consumption of soy as a possible cause.

According to the National Cancer Institute, the most prevalent cancers in U.S. children under 20 years were thyroid carcinomas (35.5 percent). There are likely many factors that are contributing to this increase, but if you or your baby have a thyroid condition, it's better to err on safety's side.

Unfortunately, if you can't breastfeed and want to avoid soy formula, there's not that much out there, assuming your baby is showing signs of lactose intolerance. Most babies can handle the hydrolized, predigested milk proteins in cow-based formula, but a few are too sensitive for even that. Therefore, a nonmilk, non-soy-based formula is necessary, and there are very few such hypoallergenic formulas on the market. The most common ones in the United States are Nutramigen and Alimentum.

### Adding Essential Fatty Acids

Scientists, lactation consultants, and health care professionals agree that "breast is best" for a plethora of reasons, not the least of which is that breast milk contains certain fatty acids that are linked to brain and visual development. Babies who are breastfed—or babies fed a formula supplemented with DHA (docosahexaenoic acid)—score significantly better on IQ tests, studies show.

These acids are not present in most current baby formulas, although several—Enfamil, Lipil, and Similac Advance—include both DHA and another valuable fatty acid, ARA (arachidonic acid), also found in breast milk. In addition, Beech-Nut now makes a baby food, First Advantage, that's fortified with DHA.

While a diet rich in DHA and ARA won't turn an average baby into a genius, it may very well be beneficial for the development of its brain and eyes. According to a 1998 study published in *The Lancet,* babies who drank a DHA-ARA-fortified formula scored significantly better at age 10 months on a three-step mental task than babies given a regular formula.

Researchers in Dundee, Scotland, enrolled 44 babies in a randomized, four-month trial. Half of the infants were given the DHA formula, while the others drank the non-DHA variety. At 10 months, long after the babies stopped drinking the trial formulas, they were given a test: to figure out how to move a barrier, lift off a blanket, and uncover a hidden toy.

The DHA-enriched babies scored significantly higher on the tests, suggesting that DHA may have a long-term effect on mental development. A similar study at University of Milan, Italy, came to the same conclusion. There have been no known adverse reactions to the addition of DHA to baby formula.

## A Personal Note

Breastfeeding advocates may tell you to "trust that nature works," and will assure you that it's rare to be unable to produce enough milk, and if you try enough techniques (nursing vacations, herbs, etc.) you'll produce more than enough milk. Unfortunately, they are more optimistic than realistic, as they are often unaware of the impact thyroid problems can have on new mothers.

Despite being knowledgeable about hypothyroidism before I became pregnant, I was not aware of the connection to breastfeeding. I intended to breastfeed, and prior to my daughter's birth, I had read several books, gone to a La Leche meeting, had some advance training from my doula (birth attendant), and after my baby was born, had several sessions with the hospital's lactation consultant.

I felt thoroughly prepared to nurse my daughter, and after she was born, all the experts assured me that she had latched on fine and we were doing well. After a week, however, she hadn't had many wet or dirty diapers and had lost weight. I was not becoming engorged between nursings, and the lactation consultants and the doula thought my milk supply might be a bit low. Although I tried many methods for increasing my milk supply, my daughter continued to lose weight, and was fussy and crying and sleeping poorly. The breastfeeding advocates insisted that if I supplemented with formula, I could forget about breastfeeding entirely, and that I should just struggle through this "rough spot" and things would work out. At that stage, I had to trust my instincts. I did not feel comfortable about that, so when my pediatrician recommended that I add supplemental formula, I agreed. My baby immediately began gaining weight, became happier, and slept better. At that point, I also turned to pumping milk to help increase my milk supply. Despite a program of regular pumping and breastfeeding, and using the supplemental nursing system, I was able to pump less than half the milk my baby needed. It was clear that I had a low milk supply and had probably had it from the beginning.

I suspected my thyroid was out of balance. When I was tested, they discovered that I'd become hyperthyroid. My thyroid hormone dosage was readjusted, but this never resulted in a rebound in milk supply. It may have been too late to kick-start it, or there may have simply been nothing I could do to produce a full supply on my own.

Despite the low milk supply, I did manage to successfully pump some of my daughter's needed milk until she was six months old, when my supply dwindled to about an ounce a day.

If your thyroid condition prevents you from breastfeeding, please be kind to yourself, and don't add guilt to the burden of your health condition. Early on, I felt terribly guilty that my baby wasn't getting proper nutrition and thriving, and then I also felt guilty that I couldn't provide enough milk. That led me to make myself nearly crazy and exhausted by trying everything—pumping, herbs, supplemental nursing tubes, and such. But after a while, I realized I had to let go of the guilt and just do the best I could for my daughter, and that meant formula, supplemented with breast milk.

An inability to breastfeed entirely or in part is not a failure, anymore than having a thyroid condition is a failure. Don't let anyone—yourself, especially—make you feel guilty for doing the best you can for your baby and yourself.

# Chapter 10

## Perimenopause, Menopause, and Premature Ovarian Failure

> You can only perceive real beauty in a person as they get older.
> —Anouk Aimee
>
> Don't deprive me of age. I have earned it.
> —May Sarton

For most women, our forties and beyond are the time of perimenopause and menopause, when we become even more aware of fluctuations in our hormone levels and their impact on our body.

For some women, this is when thyroid disease very often appears for the first time, a not so coincidental occurrence that can make for major confusion in diagnosis and treatment. Symptoms of thyroid disease can easily be mixed up with the symptoms of hormone fluctuation common to perimenopause and menopause. Unfortunately, many women wrongly assume that their symptoms are perimenopausal, rather than the underlying, undiagnosed thyroid condition that may actually be to blame.

For women with a preexisting thyroid condition, this time can also be a challenge, because the changes that take place in the hormones are interrelated with the thyroid, and the whole system can easily be shifted out of balance. According to thyroid experts Drs. Richard and Karilee Shames:

> The symptoms of hot flashes, insomnia, irritability, palpitations, and the annoying "fuzzy thinking" so common in menopause can sometimes be the result of thyroid disease. But the greatest complexity comes when actual symptoms of menopause are simply magnified and exaggerated because of the low thyroid situation that is now coexistent with menopause. As many thyroid sufferers are aware, low thyroid makes any illness worse. And while menopause is not an illness, it can certainly begin to feel that way when symptoms of low thyroid exacerbate the already annoying laundry list of female hormone symptoms.

Delia was one of those women whose doctors were confusing her menopause symptoms with undetected thyroid disease.

> Looking back, menopause was a breeze compared to the horrible symptoms of untreated hypothyroidism. But because my thyroid problems became so much worse about the same time, I blamed everything on menopause. "I'm just tired because of menopause, my hair is falling out because of menopause, I'm gaining weight because of menopause," etc. Even my doctor agreed. "How did you *expect* to feel after menopause?" (Well, duh, I sure didn't expect to feel like *this*.) He didn't recommend HRT and never did a thyroid test. My periods came further and further apart until finally

they stopped altogether. But I hardly noticed menopause had come and gone because I was so sick from thyroid. Because my hypothyroid symptoms were severe, I ended up in bed for two years waiting to "get better." After twelve years of seeing doctors who didn't recognize the symptoms of hypothyroidism, after two unnecessary colonoscopies and blood tests for everything but thyroid, after maxing out a credit card and losing a wonderful job that took me twenty years to get, I was desperate for some help. At a little corner emergency clinic, the doctor did a TSH test—my first one—which came back 275. She said, "You're very sick." I said, "Yes, I know."

During the perimenopausal period, thyroid problems that have been under control for years can even suddenly rear up again with a host of troublesome symptoms. And again, thyroid patients may assume that their symptoms are due to the thyroid or due to perimenopause, without knowing which issue is truly the cause.

Hashimoto's and hypothyroidism patient Kassie had no trouble getting pregnant with her two children. But after childbirth, she moved right into perimenopause, and her symptoms, including weight gain, worsened.

Then I began to be tired and cold again. I got brain-foggy, hair loss, and dizzy all the time. My pulse was around 40 bpm. My normal body temperature in my teens was 99.1 but now 97.2 became my new normal. Then I began to feel like I was having the never-ending allergy or cold. My periods became eratic, and blood baths to boot. You know, prior to my forties, the anwer to everything was, "Get her a pregnancy test." I used to joke that a woman could be holding her right arm in her hand and they'd want to order one. After 40, the answer was always, "It's perimenopause." Even if you tell them you have a thyroid condition, they say "Well, you're being treated, so there is no problem." Doctors kept telling me to take off the 80 pounds, but it wouldn't budge. Of course they faulted me and my self-esteem was low enough to buy into it. At one point, I joined Weight Watchers. It was hard sitting there and watching everyone else getting smaller while I'd had a big total 3-pound loss for six months. I began eating a lot of soy, as a low points source of protein. I substituted soy for all three meals about 80 percent of the week. Well, I seemed to get sicker. My TSH kept creeping up. But as far as they were concerned I was just fine because I was within the normal range. The symptoms were in my head and I needed to stop eating so much.

Kassie finally found a new endocrinologist who specialized in thyroid, and made major lifestyle, diet, and nutritional changes. She is now feeling energetic and losing weight successfully.

## What Are Perimenopause and Menopause?

It's important to first understand what perimenopause and menopause truly are.

We hear the term menopause (also referred to as "the change" or "the change of life") used to describe the period when hormonal changes are going on and symptoms become noticeable. But technically, menopause refers to the point at which menstrual periods have stopped for a full 12 months. The point when hormones start fluctuating, and in some cases declining, actually marks the start of perimenopause, the transition period toward menopause. During perimenopause, menstruation continues, although it can be erratic.

So, when people say, "I'm going through menopause," if they are still menstruating they are actually going through perimenopause. If they've stopped having periods for at least a year, they are technically postmenopausal.

What triggers perimenopause? Over time, the ovaries' production of the hormones estrogen and progesterone begins to fluctuate. The reserve of egg follicles also starts to drop. As hormones fluctuate and egg supply dwindles, more cycles become anovulatory (no ovulation), contributing further to fluctuating hormones. The menstrual cycle can become shorter, and periods may come more frequently. Usually, this is the result of a shortened follicular phase. Because there are fewer follicles, and fewer eggs recruited each cycle, the follicular phase is shortened. The luteal phase tends to remain the same length.

As menopause approaches, levels of circulating follicle-stimulating hormone (FSH) rise dramatically, in an effort to stimulate the more resistant follicles to ovulate. At the same time, the ovaries cut back on production of estrogen.

Eventually, the stock of viable eggs is depleted, and hormone levels cannot trigger ovulation; menstruation stops and menopause occurs.

When periods stop entirely—and this can occur hormonally or due to surgical removal of the uterus and ovaries—there is a fairly dramatic drop in estrogen levels. At this point, with much lower estrogen production by the ovaries, the adrenal glands also kick in to produce some estrogen. Without a corpus luteum each month, progesterone levels also drop significantly. This is a time when some women develop an imbalance: estrogen levels are high in comparison to progesterone levels—a condition known as "estrogen dominance."

As far as timing, perimenopause typically starts around three to five years—and as long as eight years—before menopause occurs. This means that for most women, perimenopause typically starts from around age 43 to 52. It's not unusual, however, for some women to have perimenopausal symptoms starting as early as their late thirties. The most common age range at which women experience hormonal menopause is 48 to 55 years, with the average age of menopause being 51 years of age. Menopause is considered late if it occurs in a woman older than 55 years.

If significant perimenopause and erratic menstruation occur substantially prior to age 40, this is called premature ovarian decline (POD). If actual menopause occurs in a woman younger than 40 years, it is called premature ovarian failure (POF). These conditions are discussed later in this chapter.

Factors that affect the age at which menopause occurs include:

- Genetics, especially the age at which your mother went through menopause. If your mother had an early menopause, chances are, you will too.
- Cigarette smoking, which is known to trigger perimenopause up to two years earlier than in nonsmokers.
- Never experiencing pregnancy, which can trigger earlier menopause, as more menstrual cycles deplete the egg supply more quickly.
- Living at high altitudes, which can trigger earlier menopause.
- Body weight or poor nutrition—excessive thinness, poor diet, malnourishment—can trigger an earlier menopause.
- Chemotherapy and radiation for cancer can damage the ovaries and trigger menopause.
- Autoimmune disease can trigger POF or POD in women under 40.

• Surgery: Women who have both ovaries removed
(bilateral oophorectomy) as part of a hysterectomy go
through surgical menopause after the time of their surgery. If the uterus is taken out, but at least one ovary
remains, a woman won't have periods but she may not
go through menopause, though she's at a higher risk. In
surgical menopause, there is no perimenopause, periods
stop immediately, and hormones drop.

Women who have been treated with radioactive iodine
(RAI) for thyroid cancer may also experience earlier menopause. In 2001, Italian researchers reported that they'd found
that RAI treatment for thyroid cancer provided sufficient radiation to damage ovarian function and follicles, reducing some
women's period of fertility and triggering earlier menopause.
The patients studied were all younger than 45 when they
received their first treatment for thyroid cancer. The researchers concluded that the RAI treatment was "probably associated
with an earlier ovarian failure in thyroid cancer patients."

## Symptoms

There are a number of symptoms that occur in women in perimenopause and menopause. Some women describe perimenopause as being like "permanent PMS."

### Menstrual Irregularities

As hormone levels decline, the interval between periods can become longer or, more commonly, shorter. Flow can vary from very
light to extremely heavy. You may miss a period occasionally or
have midcycle spotting. Over time, as you get closer to menopause,
the drop in progesterone—due to anovulatory cycles—makes pe-

riods heavier and longer-lasting. This variability in cycle length, heaviness of flow, and length of the menstrual period itself are often key evidence that menopause is approaching.

Keep in mind, however, that you can still become pregnant during this period, as you may ovulate during some cycles, and your fertile period may be difficult to predict or identify.

While some bleeding irregularities can be expected during perimenopause, any significant irregular bleeding needs to be evaluated to rule out other causes, such as uterine fibroids, uterine polyps, endometrial hyperplasia, or endometrial cancer. *All* postmenopausal bleeding must be evaluated promptly by a physician.

### Hot Flashes

The majority of woman—some estimates say as many as 75 percent to 85 percent—experience what are known formally as "climacteric symptoms," but more familiarly, hot flashes and night sweats, during perimenopause, making them the most common symptoms.

Hot flashes are due to declining estrogen levels, which can cause rapid expansion of blood vessels, which in turn makes skin temperature rise. Hot flashes, which last up to a few minutes in some people, may start with a feeling of warmth that moves from the chest to the head, causing redness and flushing in the face. You may sweat profusely for a few moments, and feel nauseated, light-headed, or dizzy. A headache and a sensation of rapid heart rate or pulse rate are also common. As the hot flash subsides, you may feel chilled, as if in a "cold sweat."

Some people have hot flashes rarely; others have them as often as once an hour, day and night. Nighttime hot flashes are known as night sweats and can disrupt sleep, even waking a woman out of a deep sleep.

"Mild" hot flashes are defined by the Food and Drug Administration as occurring less than seven times a day, on average.

### Sleep Problems

Some women have difficulty sleeping because of night sweats. They may also experience exhaustion and cognitive problems due to lack of sleep, particularly if it's difficult to fall back to sleep after awakening.

Other women experience insomnia during perimenopause, and find it difficult to fall asleep.

### Mood Changes

Much like the mechanism in PMS, the hormonal changes during perimenopause can cause irritability, mood swings, and difficulty concentrating. Exhaustion due to sleep problems can also compound these mood-related symptoms.

### Vaginal and Bladder Problems

As estrogen levels drop, the tissues lining the vagina and the vulva become drier, thinner, and less elastic. The ability to produce lubrication is affected, and this can make sexual intercourse painful for some women. The dryness can also cause burning or itching, and make women more susceptible to vaginal infections. You may also notice a change in vaginal discharge. Women also tend to lose some pelvic tone, and this can result in prolapse (a drop) of the reproductive or urinary tract organs. Symptoms of prolapse include a feeling of pressure in the vagina and pain or pressure in the lower back.

A low estrogen level also thins out the lining to the opening of the bladder—the urethra. This can put you at risk of urinary incontinence, urinary and bladder infections, and cystitis. Symptoms include frequent urination, urinary urgency, burning on urination, or an inability to urinate.

Therese describes her symptoms since going through menopause.

> My total body hormones are really messed up. Emotionally, I feel sad for about five days each month, as if I was having a menstrual cycle. I can be working on something and tears just for no reason begin running. I wake up with night sweats. I have to go to the bathroom at least twice per night. I don't take anything because I'm afraid it will mess me up even more. *Sheesh!* What a dilemma! Since I am now 58 I should be over the menopausal symptoms, but am not.

### Decreasing Fertility

As ovulation becomes less regular, your ability to conceive dramatically decreases. After the age of 40, fertility declines by at least 50 percent in most women, and the risk of miscarriage is two to three times that of younger women. (Note, however, that as long as you are having periods, and until you've hit the menopause point of 12 months without a period, it's still possible for you to become pregnant, so if you don't want to be pregnant, use birth control during this time.)

### Loss of Sex Drive

During perimenopause, sex drive can drop, and the ability to become aroused may also suffer. The cause is often hormonal.

In particular, declines in testosterone tend to have an effect on a woman's sex drive.

## Weight Change and Body Redistribution

Women gain, on average, about 5 pounds during the transition to menopause, all other things being equal. Weight is also often redistributed, as fat from hips and thighs migrates into the waist and abdominal areas, breasts lose muscle and gain fat (which contributes to sagging), and overall muscle mass decreases.

## Hair Changes

Hair on the head may thin somewhat in response to the hormonal drops. And changes in the estrogen-testosterone balance may trigger development of coarse hairs on the chin, upper lip, chest, and abdomen.

## Skin Changes

Lower estrogen reduces the skin's collagen levels, making it thinner and less elastic. Wrinkles can become more visible, and dryness of skin can contribute to the aging appearance of skin. Adult acne may worsen during this time because of hormonal fluctuations.

## Bone Loss

Women typically are at peak bone density in the 25 to 30 range. From that point on, bone loss typically occurs, at an average rate of approximately 0.13 percent per year. Perimenopause speeds up the loss to around 3 percent per year. Later, the loss steadies at around 2 percent per year. Bone loss increases your risk of osteoporosis.

### Changing Cholesterol Levels

As estrogen levels drop, some women have an increase in low-density lipoprotein (LDL) cholesterol—the "bad" cholesterol—as well as total cholesterol. This contributes to an increased risk of heart disease.

### Depression

Depression is not uncommon during perimenopause. It may be a primary symptom of hormonal changes or secondary to issues such as sleep disruption or fatigue. Care should be taken to identify mild depression, versus a clinical depression that would warrant treatment with antidepressants.

### Other Symptoms

Other symptoms of perimenopause and the menopausal transition include:

- Bloating, swollen ankles and feet
- Food cravings
- Headaches
- General fatigue or lack of energy
- Body aches and pains, backache, leg cramps
- Sagging, tender, or lumpy breasts
- Facial hair
- Heart palpitations

## Testing

Testing isn't always done to officially diagnose perimenopause or menopause. Typically, symptoms in a younger woman who has a regular menstrual cycle are more likely to be the result of premenstrual syndrome than perimenopause. Irregular cycles and symptoms in a woman 40 and older point to perimenopause. And the lack of menstrual periods for a year is considered evidence of menopause in a woman over 40.

In some cases, however, blood testing is done to help pinpoint declining hormones; most often, follicle-stimulating hormone (FSH) will be tested. The closer to menopause, the more these levels will increase.

Around the time of menopause, many practitioners also recommend bone density testing. The recommended test to evaluate bone loss (osteoporosis) is the DEXA (dual-energy X-ray absorptiometry) scan, which evaluates bone mineral density. Some practitioners do a preliminary scan of bone density in the heel, which is considered a screening and not diagnostic test.

## Menopause or Thyroid Disease?

According to the American Association of Clinical Endocrinologists, millions of women suffering a variety of unresolved symptoms thought to be menopause-related—even some who receive estrogen replacement therapies for menopausal symptoms—are actually suffering from undiagnosed thyroid disease. The two conditions often develop in women at the same general age, and they often appear at the same time as well. In addition, they share many common symptoms.

The AACE survey reported a disturbing statistic: "Only one in four women who have discussed menopause with a physician were recommended to be tested for thyroid disease."

Perhaps as surprising, one-third of women 40 years of age and older surveyed did not even discuss menopause at all with their physicians!

Take a look at Table 4, which outlines the common symptoms of menopause and lines them up against common symptoms of hypothyroidism and hyperthyroidism.

It's easy to see that almost all of the symptoms commonly assumed to be menopause, except for vaginal and bladder problems, and sagging or tender breasts, can in fact be due to an undiagnosed thyroid condition. This is why some experts believe that all women with menopausal symptoms should be thoroughly evaluated for underlying thyroid disorder.

Getting proper evaluation and diagnosis may be more difficult for a women approaching menopause, as fluctuating hormones may make the standard thyroid tests less reliable. According to Drs. Richard and Karilee Shames:

> One way out of this testing dilemma is to have your doctor order thyroid antibodies tests in addition to TSH, free T-3 and free T-4 tests, which may serve as a better indicator of your actual status. Anything suspicious with these tests, in our opinion, warrants a trial of thyroid hormone. This is our opinion regardless of whether the woman in question is already on hormone replacement therapy or is simply contemplating it.

In women where there is a high suspicion of thyroid disease, but the traditional tests show normal results, the TRH test, discussed in Chapter 3, is recommended for more in-depth evaluation of thyroid function.

## TABLE 4. COMPARISON OF SYMPTOMS IN (PERI) MENOPAUSE AND THYROID DISORDERS

| Symptom | (Peri) Menopause | Hypothyroidism | Hyperthyroidism |
|---|---|---|---|
| Menstrual irregularities | X | X | X |
| Hot flashes | X | | X |
| Sleep problems | X | X | X |
| Mood changes | X | X | X |
| Vaginal/bladder problems | X | | |
| Decreased fertility | X | X | X |
| Loss of sex drive | X | X | X |
| Weight gain | X | X | X |
| Muscle mass loss | X | X | X |
| Hair loss | X | X | X |
| Skin changes | X | X | X |
| Bone loss | X | X | X |
| Changing cholesterol levels | X | X | X |
| Depression | X | X | X |
| Bloating, swollen feet | X | X | X |
| Food cravings | X | X | X |
| Headaches | X | X | X |
| Fatigue, lack of energy | X | X | X |
| Body aches and pains | X | X | X |
| Sagging, tender breasts | X | | |
| Heart palpitations | X | X | X |

## Does Menopause Need "Treatment"?

There's no question that modern medicine has turned menopause into a disease, and views it as a negative, a time of decline and deterioration of the reproductive system and hormone levels. But naturopathic doctor and hormone educator Sherrill Sellman cautions against this view.

Menopause is not a downhill slide nor an "estrogen deficiency disease" as the medical world likes to call it. At menopause there is an adjustment in estrogen levels, reducing the output by the ovaries by about 40–60 percent. Just low enough so that the menopausal woman won't be maturing eggs. Nature has also provided a backup system in the estrogen department—both the fat cells and the adrenals produce estrogen. If we have any "meat on our bones," menopausal women are generally making plenty of estrogen, even if they have had a full hysterectomy!

However, with menopause there is a cessation of ovulation. When we ovulate, the site, known as a follicle, from which an eggs bursts forth turns into an endocrine gland that makes progesterone. When there's no ovulation, the primary supply of progesterone is not available. Thus, there is a precipitous fall in progesterone levels at menopause. However, once again, nature's backup system makes progesterone from the adrenals.

Many women navigate perimenopause and menopause without additional symptoms and don't require treatment. Other women find that the symptoms do become problematic, and for these women, it's important to identify the cause of the problems, which may include:

- An underlying thyroid problem
- Estrogen deficiency
- Progesterone deficiency
- Estrogen dominance: too much estrogen in relation to progesterone
- Adrenal fatigue or burnout
- Onset of autoimmune disease

The testing and evaluation of these symptoms are discussed in Chapter 11.

## Hormone Therapies

Hormone therapy seeks to regulate hormonal shifts, which can help minimize or eliminate perimenopausal or menopausal symptoms. Typically, the hormonal treatments contain estrogen or progesterone alone, or a combination of estrogen plus synthetic progesterone known as progestin.

### Oral Contraceptives

Oral contraceptives are often the treatment of choice to relieve perimenopausal symptoms—even if you don't need them for birth control.

Today's low-dose pills regulate periods and may eliminate or reduce hot flashes, vaginal dryness, and premenstrual syndrome. Brand names of the some of the lower-dose pills that include both estrogen and progestins are: Alesse, Levlite, Loestrin, Mircette, and Ortho Evra.

Oral contraceptives regulate hormones, which can reduce some of the perimenopausal symptoms that stem from fluctuations. In addition, they can help preserve fertility, may protect against uterine and ovarian cancers, and may reduce acne. Oral contraceptives do have risks: they raise the risk of heart attack and stroke and are particularly dangerous to women over 35 and women who smoke.

Progestin-only pills—known as the "mini-pill"—are considered safer for women over 35, women who smoke, have high blood pressure, are overweight, or have a history of blood clots. Brand names include Micronor, Nor-QD, and Ovrette.

## Conventional Hormone Replacement Therapy

For decades, estrogen (available by prescription either with or without synthetic progesterone, called progestin) has been the primary treatment for perimenopausal and menopausal symptoms. These treatments were considered particularly effective for hot flashes and night sweats, and also to protect against osteoporosis.

Estrogen therapy

- Effectively treats hot flashes
- Helps reduce the risk of osteoporosis by building bone mass and reducing the risk of fractures
- Improves cholesterol
- Helps with urinary symptoms
- Treats vaginal symptoms
- May help reduce the risk of colorectal cancer
- May help prevent Alzheimer's disease.

Estrogens given as medication can be naturally derived or synthetic. Estrogen is available in a variety of forms, including:

- Skin patches (Vivelle, Climara, Estraderm, Esclim, Alora)
- Creams (such as Estrace, Estrasorb, a cream to be applied to legs and thighs, and Premarin cream)
- Gel (Estrogel)
- Oral tablets (Premarin, Cenestin, Estratab, Ortho-Est, and Estinyl)
- Vaginal rings, suppositories, and creams, such as Estring and Femring, which are mainly useful for vaginal symptoms

For a woman who still has a uterus, taking estrogen alone (known as "unopposed estrogen") increases the risk of getting endometrial cancer, a cancer of the uterine lining, due to chronic estrogen stimulation. Adding progestin helps protect the uterus and lowers this risk.

Estrogen-progestin combinations are also available in products such as the Combipatch and Ortho-Prefest skin patches, Femhrt tablets, Activella, and Prempro/Premphase tablets.

### Dangers of HRT

In 1991, the National Heart, Lung, and Blood Institute and other units of the National Institutes of Health launched the Women's Health Initiative, one of the largest studies of its kind ever undertaken in the United States, looking at more than 160,000 women. Both hormone studies were to have continued until 2005, but were stopped early; the estrogen-plus-progestin study was halted in July 2002, and the estrogen-alone study at the end of February 2004. The findings were significant.

1. Estrogen alone (i.e., Premarin) raises the risk of blood clots and stroke.
2. The dangers of estrogen-progestin combination therapy include increased risk of
   - Blood clots
   - Stroke
   - Heart attacks
   - Breast cancer (and harder-to-detect tumors)
   - Gallbladder disease
   - Dementia

Many practitioners and patients are reluctant to use traditional hormone replacement therapy, given the risks. In general, though, the absolute risk to each particular woman is still considered quite low.

Some doctors will still prescribe estrogen, or an estrogen-progestin combination, for some women with a low cancer risk, but a high risk of osteoporosis and debilitating menopause symptoms. For these women, the benefits of short-term therapy are considered greater than the risk.

Generally, however, a woman should take the lowest possible effective dose, for the shortest amount of time. And keep in mind, if you have only vaginal symptoms, you should look for a locally applied product, such as a vaginal cream or ring, rather than one taken by mouth or absorbed through the skin, which enters the bloodstream.

### Bioidentical Hormone Replacement Therapy

Bioidentical hormones are a new way to approach hormone replacement and may help resolve various perimenopausal and menopausal symptoms. They are discussed in detail in Chapter 11.

### Estrogen, Phytoestrogens, and Hypothyroidism Treatment

According to a study reported in 2001 in the *New England Journal of Medicine*, women with hypothyroidism who are taking thyroid hormone replacement medication may need an increased dosage if they begin estrogen treatment after menopause. In the study conducted by endocrinologist Baha Arafah, of University Hospitals of Cleveland, he found that the additional thyroid medicine needed was "small but potentially clinically important" when women began taking the estrogen to relieve menopausal symptoms. According to Dr. Arafah, hypothyroidism worsens in as many as 40 percent of thyroid patients beginning estrogen treatment for menopause. In a related editorial, Robert D. Utiger, M.D., states his conclusion, that:

> Because women with hypothyroidism who are taking thyroxine may need more thyroxine when they are treated with estrogen and may need less thyroxine after estrogen is discontinued, it is prudent to reassess their thyroid function several months after estrogen therapy is either initiated or discontinued.

Even women who are using a lot of phytoestrogens, such as those found in soy foods, should be rechecked as well.

Generally, it's advised that women on thyroid hormone treatment have comprehensive thyroid levels evaluated no more than 12 weeks after they begin estrogen or phytoestrogen therapy, to determine if an increase in thyroid dosage is needed.

Even if blood tests are normal, some physicians suggest that if thyroid symptoms worsen after starting estrogen or phytoestrogen treatment, you need a slight dosage increase to account for the binding effect on thyroid hormone not measurable in the tests.

## Other Drugs

### Antidepressants

Antidepressants can be helpful with some symptoms, including hot flashes, mood changes, and depression. Some studies have shown that the antidepressant venlafaxine (Effexor) may actually decrease hot flashes by up to 60 percent. The anti-depressants known as selective serotonin reuptake inhibitors (SSRIs)—including paroxetine (Paxil), fluoxetine (Prozac/Sara-fem), sertraline (Zoloft), and citalopram (Celexa)—are also being tested and show some evidence of being able to help relieve hot flashes. These medications can have some unwanted side effects, however, including nausea, dizziness, or sexual dysfunction.

## Drugs for Hot Flashes

Some women find that hot flashes respond to the drug gaba-pentin, known by its brand name Neurontin. While it's actu-ally a drug used for seizures and nerve pain, it has been shown to reduce hot flashes. It does have side effects in some people, however: drowsiness, dizziness, nausea, and swelling.

Another drug for hot flashes is clonidine (Catapres). This high blood pressure drug, available in a pill and patch form, may help reduce the frequency of hot flashes. It does have side effects in some people: dizziness, drowsiness, dry mouth, and constipation.

The drug belladonna (Bellergal) can help some women with hot flashes, but due to its addictive properties, it's not used very often, and even then, only for a short period.

## Osteoporosis Drugs

While the hormone replacement drugs used to be prescribed to help protect against osteoporosis, other drugs are now being given to women during menopause.

Bisphosphonates—nonhormonal bisphosphonate medi-cations, including alendronate (Fosamax) and risedronate (Actonel)—can reduce bone loss and help reduce the risk of bone fractures. They are the most popular treatment for osteoporosis. Side effects can include nausea, stomach pain, and esophageal irritation and pain that may also pose an increased risk of ulcers.

Selective estrogen receptor modulators (SERMs) include raloxifene (Evista), which, while not a hormone, mimics the effects of estrogen on bone density in postmenopausal women, but without the increased breast and uterine cancer risks. Raloxifene's most common side effect, however, is hot flashes. It is also not recommended for anyone with a history or risk of blood clots.

Calcitonin (Miacalcin or Calcimar) is a hormone, delivered by nasal spray or injection, that may help reduce some fracture risk and slow bone loss in women with osteoporosis. It helps maintain bone density but is not as potent or effective as bisphosphonates for treating osteoporosis. However, calcitonin does sometimes help relieve pain in women who already have compression fractures due to osteoporosis.

Teriparatide (Forteo) is a recently approved drug that is derived from parathyroid hormone. Given once a day by injection to the thigh or abdomen, Teriparatide is for postmenopausal women with a high fracture risk. The drug stimulates new bone growth, leading to increased bone mineral density. Animal studies showed increased risk of cancer, so the drug carries a black-box warning regarding cancer risks. Mild side effects can occur, including nausea, dizziness, fast heart beats, and leg cramps.

Some doctors recommend progesterone therapy to control hot flashes.

## Self-Care

Self-care can help prevent and help you cope with hot flashes. Even a slight increase in body temperature can trigger hot flashes, so one thing you can do is to stay cool, as much as you can. This may mean dressing more lightly, or in layers, so that you can quickly remove clothing if you feel too warm. You may also want to turn the thermostat down or open windows during colder weather, and use air conditioning or fans during warmer weather. You may want to sleep in light, natural fiber clothing that breathes, on cotton sheets, with your bedroom cooler, to avoid night sweats. If you feel a hot flash coming on, try sipping a cold drink. You'll also want to learn, and then avoid, your particular hot flash triggers. For many women, these include hot drinks, spicy or very hot foods, alcohol, and hot weather or a warm room.

### Diet

Increased heart disease risk means that it's particularly important to adopt a healthier diet, focusing on low-fat, high-fiber vegetables and fruits rich in nutrients. The increased risk of osteoporosis calls for an increase in calcium-rich foods and the addition of a calcium supplement. Cut back on calories if hormonal changes are contributing to weight gain.

Pay attention to which foods trigger hot flashes and stay away from the common culprits, which can include spicy hot dishes, caffeine, and alcohol.

### Exercise

Exercise is one of the best ways to help deal with perimenopausal and menopausal symptoms, as exercise can help elevate mood, reduce stress, combat fatigue and depression, strengthen bones, improve sleep, and ward off hormonally related weight gain. Try to exercise for 30 minutes or more on most days of the week. Some studies have shown that exercise can help reduce hot flashes, palpitations, and some of the other perimeno-pausal and menopausal symptoms.

You may also want to do exercises to help strengthen the pelvic floor muscle. These exercises, known as Kegel exercises, can help with some menopausal-related urinary incontinence.

### Stress Reduction

Stress reduction is critical, and should be practiced as a regular part of your overall approach to good health. Find the stress reducer that works best for you. It may be prayer, meditation, yoga, acupuncture, hypnosis, biofeedback, deep-breathing exercises, or guided visualizations and imagery. Even if they don't affect your menopause symptoms directly, these techniques help ensure better sleep and less fatigue.

### Paced Respiration

One particularly effective stress reduction technique for meno-pause is known as paced respiration or paced breathing. This is a technique of slow, deep breathing. In one study, paced respiration, when done twice daily, actually decreased the frequency of hot flashes by 50 percent over a four-month study period. Other studies of paced respiration have shown that women who practice it also have lower average skin temperature, which is a means of measuring hot flashes.

Paced respiration is not hard, but it takes some practice. It's a diaphragmatic breathing technique, which means you need to keep your rib cage still, and inhale and exhale using your stomach muscles to lower and raise your diaphragm. You can try it yourself.

- Start by sitting in a comfortable, quiet place.
- Inhale for five seconds, without moving your rib cage.
- Exhale for five seconds, pulling your stomach muscles in and up.
- Repeat this cycle of breathing.

To practice, spend 10 to 15 minutes twice a day. When you feel a hot flash coming on, stop whatever you are doing, find a quiet place, and perform paced respiration until the hot flash subsides. You may even be able to prevent the hot flash from developing. A few minutes of paced respiration can also help calm stress during a hectic day.

### Stop Smoking

If you smoke, stopping smoking is one of the most important things you can do to help relieve symptoms, not to mention improve your health, while reducing the risk of many serious health conditions such as heart disease, stroke, cancer, and lung disease. Cigarette smoking is linked to both earlier menopause and hot flashes.

### Vaginal Discomforts

If you have vaginal discomfort, such as dryness or discomfort with intercourse, you may want to try an over-the-counter water-based vaginal lubricant such as Astroglide or K-Y Jelly, or a vaginal moisturizer like Replens or Vagisil. Some experts also recommend staying sexually active!

*Optimize Sleep*

Make sure that you are getting sufficient quality sleep. Sufficient means seven to eight hours a night for most people. And quality means that you are staying asleep, without frequent waking, and reaching deep, restorative sleep. You may want to avoid caffeinated drinks and vigorous exercise before bedtime. Relaxation techniques, including breathing, guided imagery or relaxation, progressive muscle relaxation, or meditation can help achieve deeper, more refreshing sleep.

## Alternative and Natural Treatments

### *Phytoestrogens and Isoflavones*

Soy and red clover are both sources of isoflavones, which are plant-derived compounds that occur in certain foods that act somewhat like estrogen in the body. Isoflavones are typically found in soybeans, chickpeas, and other legumes. Some experts believe that isoflavones, and soy in particular, can help with menopausal symptoms. Because women in Asian countries, who regularly have soy in their diet, have fewer hot flashes and menopausal symptoms it was thought that soy might be a treatment. Most formal studies, however, have found isoflavones are generally ineffective in relieving menopause symptoms.

Despite the myths that prevail, Asians actually do not eat large quantities of soy. Rather, the typical Asian diet may include 5 to 10 grams of soy protein per day. This is in contrast to some American diets, which may include as much as 60 grams of soy protein a day, from various processed forms of soy, soy supplements, soy milk, and so on.

When taken as a food in its fermented form—as tempeh or miso and not overconsumed, soy appears to be safe. When overconsumed, or used as a dietary supplement for longer periods of time, however, soy has been associated with thickening of the uterus, thyroid dysfunction, menstrual disruption, fertility problems, and other hormonal effects.

Some controversial studies have even suggested that phytoestrogens such as soy may even promote breast cancer growth, and practitioners caution some groups of women against using phytoestrogens, especially

- Women who have had or are at increased risk for breast cancer, uterine cancer, or ovarian cancer
- Women who have had uterine fibroids
- Women taking birth control pills
- Women already taking prescription hormone replacement therapy
- Women taking cancer drugs known as selective estrogen receptor modulators (SERMs), such as tamoxifen
- Women who have had or are at increased risk of autoimmune thyroid disease or other autoimmune conditions

In an interview on my website, Dr. Sherrill Sellman, an expert on women's hormones, explained how she used to be a big fan of soy until she began to do more research.

> Now I err on the side of caution and actually advise women to cut way down on their soy intake. The most preferred kind of soy would be the fermented versions such as tempeh and miso because that is the most digestible form of soy. The fermentation process destroys the harmful toxins found in soy.... It is also a very allergic food and hard to digest.

## Dong Quai

Dong quai (*angelica sinensis*) is an herb used in Chinese medicine to help support hormonal balance. Dong quai does not have estrogen effects, so it's considered fairly safe. Women who are taking the anticoagulant drug warfarin (Coumadin) should not use dong quai, however, as there can be bleeding complications.

## Black Cohosh

The herbal supplement black cohosh is a popular supplement for menopause. While it does not act like estrogen, it is thought to help reduce hot flashes. Remifemin is a commercial menopause preparation that contains black cohosh. Many experts do not recommend using black cohosh for more than six months. In the short term, few side effects are seen, but long-term safety has not been studied. Occasionally, side effects of black cohosh can include stomach upset, vomiting, dizziness, visual disturbances, a slowed heartbeat, and sweating. Black cohosh should not be taken by a woman who is experiencing heavy bleeding.

## Ginseng

Panax ginseng is thought to help with some menopausal symptoms, such as mood symptoms and sleep disturbances, and with overall well-being. It has not been found helpful for hot flashes, however.

## Kava

Kava may decrease anxiety, but there is no evidence that it decreases hot flashes. (*Note*: The FDA has issued warnings about kava because of the herb's potential for liver damage.)

## Calcium

Typically, after menopause women should take at least 1,500 mg of calcium daily to help prevent loss of bone mineral density. Other women, including perimenopausal women, should take 1,000 to 1,200 mg daily. Ideally, calcium should be obtained from food. The following are some guidelines to calcium content.

- Milk, regular or skim, 1 cup = 300 mg calcium
- Calcium-fortified orange juice, 1 cup = 300 mg calcium
- Yogurt, regular or fat-free, 1 cup = 400 mg calcium
- Cheddar cheese, 1 ounce = about 200 mg calcium
- Salmon, 3 ounces = 200 mg calcium

It can be hard to eat enough calcium-rich foods to get sufficient amounts, so many people need calcium supplements. You can use something as simple and inexpensive as calcium carbonate (i.e., Tums), or calcium citrate supplements. Many practitioners suggest you avoid calcium products made from bone meal, dolomite, or oyster shells, as these products may contain unnecessary lead.

Since you can't absorb more than around 500 mg of calcium at a time, spread out calcium supplementation throughout the day.

If you have sarcoidosis or kidney stones, you need to talk to your practitioner before taking calcium supplements.

*Note*: If you are taking Synthroid, Armour, or any of the levothyroxine or other thyroid hormone replacement drugs, calcium can interfere with absorption of these drugs, so allow at least four hours between taking your calcium supplements and taking your thyroid hormone drugs.

## *Vitamin D*

Vitamin D is essential for calcium absorption. Approximately 400 IU for people under 70, and 600 IU for those over 70, is recommended.

## *DHEA*

Dehydroepiandrosterone (DHEA) is a precursor hormone that is converted to estrogen and testosterone. DHEA can be taken as a supplement. There is some anecdotal evidence that DHEA may help with hot flashes and low sex drive, but studies are still under way, and some practitioners are concerned about long-term effects of DHEA.

Most experts agree that you should not self-treat with DHEA. Instead, ask your practitioner to do a blood test to evaluate DHEA-sulfate (DHEA-S) levels. If your levels are borderline or low, you may want to try low-dose DHEA supplementation with a high-quality DHEA.

## *Essential Fatty Acids*

Essential fatty acids are the "good fats" that your body needs, but cannot make itself, so you must get them from food or supplements. Essential fatty acids help synthesize prostaglandins, which can help reduce inflammation, boost immune function, decrease menstrual cramps, and fight PMS and menopausal symptoms. They can also reduce your risk of heart disease by helping control blood pressure and reducing the risk of atherosclerosis.

Two oils in particular—evening primrose oil and flaxseed (either as an oil or in the seed form)—deliver omega-3 fatty acids, which are particularly helpful for women. While they have no reported effects on hot flashes, evening primrose oil and flaxseed have been tested and shown to help with PMS and cramps, irritability, headaches, skin, water retention, hair loss, and breast pain, and they can boost the immune system. These oils can also help maintain moisture in skin, hair, vaginal issue, and other mucous membranes.

The essential fatty acid found in fish and fish oil supplements also has protective value for the heart and may help reduce inflammation.

Researchers have also found that by maintaining the proper balance of dietary fats, a substantial amount of the bone loss associated with the postmenopausal period may be avoided. Diets with a lower ratio of omega-6 fatty acids (fats found in grains and beef), compared to omega-3 fatty acids (fats found in plants, nuts, fish) may minimize bone loss. The mechanism behind this is that estrogen blocks particular inflammatory compounds that prevent bone formation. So, when estrogen levels fall after menopause, osteoporosis can worsen because these inflammatory compounds are not blocked. Omega-3 fatty acids may reduce the body's ability to produce these inflammatory compounds, which in turn helps protect bone.

### Maca

New York–based anthropologist Viana Muller has been making trips to Peru since 1989, exploring both the rain forest and the Andes in search of effective herbal remedies unknown to North Americans. One of the most promising native remedies that Dr. Muller has studied is maca, a cruciferous root from the same botanical family as the turnip and broccoli. Maca grows at 12,500 to 14,500 feet above sea level in the high Andean plateaus of central Peru, making it the highest-growing food plant in the world. Maca is believed to be one of the earliest domesticated food plants of Peru, right along with the potato.

According to Dr. Muller:

> The root of the maca plant has been used successfully for centuries by the native people of Peru. They use it for various medicinal purposes, such as enhancing fertility in people and animals, improving hormonal balance, increasing sex drive, reducing hot flashes and vaginal dryness, regulating menstrual problems, and enhancing energy.

Maca is rich in essential minerals, especially selenium, calcium, magnesium, and iron, and includes linolenic, palmitic, and oleic fatty acids and polysaccharides. Maca is an adaptogen, which means it helps the body adapt to stress and seeks to balance, rather than supplement, the hormonal system.

Native medicine practitioners and herbalists have recommended maca for a number of purposes.

- To reduce or eliminate menopausal symptoms, such as hot flashes, vaginal dryness, and hormone-related depression, as an alternative to hormone replacement therapy (HRT)
- To provide nutritional support for the endocrine system, including the adrenals, the thyroid, the ovaries, and the testes
- To regulate and normalize menstrual cycles
- To promote healthy fertility in both men and women
- To promote healthy libido and erectile function

- To support a healthy immune system without overstimulating the immune system or endangering people with autoimmune disease
- To increase energy, stamina, and endurance

Research has shown that maca contains no plant hormones, unlike soy. Instead, its action relies on plant sterols, which act as chemical triggers to help the body itself produce a higher level of hormone appropriate to the age and gender of the person taking it.

According to Dr. Muller, maca works through the pituitary, helping to balance all of the endocrine and reproductive glands. High-potency organic maca root also appears to have powerful beneficial effects on the immune system.

> The alkaloids in the maca root stimulate the hypothalamus and pituitary to produce more precursor hormones which then impact all of the endocrine glands—the pineal, the adrenals, ovaries, testes, pancreas, and the thyroid gland. So maca appears to be stimulating the body to produce its own hormones more adequately rather than supplying hormones from an outside source.

Since introducing maca to the United States in the 1990s, Dr. Muller has seen a dramatic increase in the use of this medicinal herb by holistic practitioners in the United States. While maca is a cruciferous vegetable, the fact that maca supplements are precooked removes any goitrogenic properties for thyroid patients.

*Note*: The quality of maca available for sale varies widely. Inexpensive maca is almost always poorly produced. Only certified organic maca has been extensively tested and shown to be effective.

## *Other Supplements*

Other recommended supplements to help with perimenopausal and menopausal symptoms include:

- A good-quality multivitamin
- Magnesium, 500 to 1000 mg before sleeping
- A high potency B-complex vitamin
- Vitamin E, 400 IU daily
- Zinc, 15 to 50 mg daily

## The Osteoporosis-Thyroid Controversy

There are some inconclusive studies that have shown that hyperthyroidism or suppressed, extremely low TSH levels, can be a risk factor for osteoporosis. At the same time, there are many reputable studies that find no significant reduction in bone mass in people on thyroid hormone replacement, even when at levels that result in a suppressed TSH, hence no increased risk of osteoporosis.

While the research is contradictory, some doctors have only focused on the osteoporosis risk and use this information as an argument against treating menopausal women for mild or subclinical hypothyroidism.

Some doctors compound the problem by employing faulty logic: if a very low TSH level poses a risk, then when treating perimenopausal and menopausal hypothyroid women, why not keep them at higher levels, and thereby avoid the risk? Hence, the current penchant on the part of some doctors to medicate only to high-normal TSH levels, leaving these women only partially treated for hypothyroidism. These women then walk around feeling unwell, being told it's menopause and not their thyroid, with the doctor refusing to prescribe a higher dose of thyroid hormone.

According to Drs. Richard and Karilee Shames, thyroid hormone is not the osteoporosis villain that it has been painted to be in the past.

> The controversy started some years ago when research data on bone density and menopausal women was beginning to be collected. The results seemed to suggest that thyroid hormone treatment was associated with a lowered bone density. Both doctors and patients alike became fearful of thyroxine, and tried to treat even overt hypothyroidism with as little medicine as possible. This resulted in many people receiving a dose too low to relieve their symptoms, but it was considered a worthy tradeoff. Patients were told they would have to continue suffering through some low thyroid symptoms now in order to preserve their bone density for the future. However, the studies at that time lacked the data available today from third-generation TSH assays and high-resolution bone densitometry. In addition, the groups of patients then being analyzed lacked the diversity necessary for accurate study. With further research now pouring in, it appears clear that thyroid medication—even in the higher doses some people need to feel best—does not increase one's fracture risk in later years.

One late 2003 review looked at 63 English-language studies of the thyroid-osteoporosis connection that were published from 1990 to 2001. Of the 63 studies reviewed, levothyroxine was shown to have no overall effect in 31 studies; partial positive and/or partial negative effects were reported in 23 studies; only 9 studies showed overall negative effects; and 3 studies reported no effects at all.

Ultimately, this meta-review found no association between the duration of levothyroxine therapy and an associated reduction of bone mineral density, if it occurs. There was no conclusive evidence of a dose-effect relationship when all studies were considered. Not surprisingly, age-specific effects of levothyroxine on bone mineral density loss were reported by these studies, with older women experiencing the greatest effects. In those studies where some negative impact was postulated, the adverse effects of levothyroxine on bone mineral density were reported to be greater in postmenopausal than in premenopausal women. Even then, it wasn't clear whether underlying thyroid diseases and/or their treatments were simply additional risk factors for women already at risk of osteoporosis. In general, the reviewers conclude that all of the current evidence considered together suggests no significant effect of levothyroxine on bone mineral density, but caution that this is a preliminary conclusion, and more studies should be done.

Say the Shames:

It makes no sense to soft-peddle thyroid hormone treatment in the face of this new evidence. Careful research in the last few years indicates that proper doses of thyroid medication do not increase fracture risk.

If you have a family history of osteoporosis and are on thyroid hormone replacement, or you are postmenopausal and on thyroid hormone replacement—and particularly if you have a history of hyperthyroidism or Graves' disease—you should be screened for risk factors of osteoporosis, have bone densitometry testing if warranted, receive counseling on diet and exercise, and receive prescriptions for osteotherapeutic drugs, if warranted.

Other practitioners suggest you also add 1,500 to 2,000 mg of a highly absorbable bone-friendly calcium supplement daily (but remember not to take them within four hours of your thyroid hormone replacement drugs), eat mineral rich foods, and consider supplementing with a trace mineral product.

## Premature Ovarian Decline, Premature Ovarian Failure, Primary Ovarian Insufficiency

Some women experience what used to be called "premature menopause," but is now referred to by new terms: premature ovarian decline (POD), premature ovarian failure (POF), or primary ovarian insufficiency (POI).

In premature ovarian decline the ovaries are not functioning optimally long before menopause or perimenopause would typically occur. POD in some cases leads to premature ovarian failure, where ovaries stop normal functioning entirely.

In POD and POF, there are anovulatory cycles, and many women have either a low supply of follicles or follicles that are not viable. Follicle-stimulating hormone levels are also typically elevated, as there is an attempt to stimulate the ovaries into ovulating regularly. While this elevated FSH is normal in women who are perimenopausal or menopausal, in women with POD and POF, the elevated FSH occurs much earlier—as early as the teens in some women, and more frequently in the twenties and thirties. The official definition of POD or POF, however, is a slowdown or complete cessation of ovarian function before the age of 40.

POD and POF are considered in large part to be autoimmune conditions, and women with autoimmune thyroid disease—Hashimoto's or Graves' disease—are therefore at higher risk of having the antiovarian antibodies and autoimmune oophoritis (inflammation of the ovaries) that often is a cause of POD and POF.

Some experts characterize the four stages of this condition, as follows:

- Stage 1. A woman has *normal* FSH levels, is unable to become pregnant, and fails to respond to FSH therapy for superovulation (Pergonal).
- Stage 2. A woman has *elevated* FSH levels, is unable to become pregnant, and fails to respond during FSH therapy for superovulation.
- Stage 3. A woman has elevated FSH levels, with menstrual irregularities.
- Stage 4. A woman's menstrual periods have stopped entirely.

The most common early symptom is almost always irregular menstrual periods. The other symptoms of POD and POF are similar to perimenopause and menopause—they just occur much earlier: infertility, hot flashes and night sweats, irritability, difficulty concentrating, low sex drive, vaginal dryness, pain during intercourse, and complete cessation of periods.

Some experts estimate that as many as 5 percent of young women experience three months without a menstrual period each year, yet only 40 percent of these women get a medical evaluation for this problem. One of the challenges is that doctors frequently prescribe an oral contraceptive to help regulate the menstrual cycle, without identifying the underlying problem, or determining that the woman has POD/POF/POI. The woman may then take the contraceptive pill for years and progress to stage 4, beyond a point where intervention in the form of fertility treatments may have permitted pregnancy.

As many as 10 to 20 percent of women will have a family history of POD/POF, but in many cases, there is no clear reason for it. Key risk factors, however, include chemotherapy, radiation, bone marrow transplant, exposure to certain toxins and solvents, chromosomal or genetic issues, cigarette smoking, and viral and autoimmune attack on the ovaries (oophoritis). These various irregularities can cause lower-than-normal follicles or a dysfunction in the follicles and ovaries.

We do know that these conditions appear to be more common in women with thyroid conditions, especially hypothyroidism. One study found that 27 percent of women with POF also had low thyroid function. In some women, there is underlying autoimmune oophoritis, in which the immune system targets the ovaries themselves, causing inflammation and gradually making them unable to function. Antibodies testing can identify the antiovarian antibodies that diagnose oophoritis. Other autoimmune disorders also seen in association with POD/POF include Graves' disease, Sjögren syndrome, rheumatoid arthritis, and vitiligo.

In POD and POF, a woman isn't making enough estrogen and progesterone. In POD, and in milder cases of POF, hormone replacement therapy may help, and there are a few reports that high-dose corticosteroid treatment may induce ovulation in some women, but this is a controversial treatment.

It is frequently difficult for women with POD and POF to become pregnant, because ovaries are not functioning properly and hormone levels are insufficient.

To diagnose POD or POF, your doctor will typically measure the levels of FSH in your bloodstream. Since FSH is the trigger that readies eggs for ovulation, high FSH can be a sign of ovarian dysfunction. In addition, serum prolactin, luteinizing hormone (LH), and estradiol should be measured.

Even among women with full POF, as many as 5 to 10 percent still become pregnant without treatment, due to apparent spontaneous remission of their condition, even years after diagnosis. At present, researchers aren't able to predict which women will have such a remission or explain why it occurs.

Hormone replacement therapy may help with POD and POF. Unlike menopause-related HRT—found to increase the risk of stroke, blood clots, heart disease, heart attacks, and breast cancer—many experts believe that replacing hormones to natural age-appropriate levels in women who have documented hormone deficiencies does not carry significant risks.

# Part III

# FINDING SOLUTIONS

## Chapter 11

# Creating Your Own Thyroid Hormone Breakthrough

*When people tell you you can't do something, you kind of want to try it.*

—Margaret Chase Smith

Whatever hormonal health challenge you may be facing—PMS, fertility challenges, menstrual problems, low sex drive, a problem pregnancy, or a difficult menopause—the most important thing you can do is get your thyroid function tested properly and thoroughly. As an empowered patient, it will be your responsibility to ensure that you have the right practitioner who performs the right tests.

If you do have a thyroid condition—be it a subclinical condition, hypothyroidism or hyperthyroidism, or even the presence of autoimmune antibodies—you must get proper and thorough treatment.

Hopefully, this book has given you an understanding of how to get a thyroid condition diagnosed, what proper treatment involves, and the role that the thyroid plays in hormonal conditions.

In this closing chapter, I've summarized some of the key recommendations that can help you in your journey toward good health!

## Don't Take No for an Answer When It Comes to Getting Tested

It's unfortunate, but doctors sometimes don't take women's complaints seriously. Instead of looking for physical causes of our symptoms, some physicians are hard-wired into the idea that intangible symptoms—fatigue, sleep problems, anxiety, depression, for example—are evidence of a mental health condition. It's simpler to just hand over an antidepressant prescription than to do the detective work necessary to determine whether a woman has an underlying thyroid condition, estrogen dominance, excess cortisol, or other hormonal imbalance that may be causing these "mental" symptoms.

But after nearly a decade as a patient advocate, and having talked to or corresponded with thousands of women, there is one thing I am quite certain about: women usually know their bodies. We can be very tuned in. When we know that something is "not quite right," and we're pretty sure that it's not a mental health problem, we're almost always correct.

In this country we have an epidemic of undiagnosed and misdiagnosed thyroid disease. So trust your instincts and trust yourself. If you suspect that difficulty getting pregnant is more than just "anxiety" and a question of "take your time," go ahead and push for further testing. If your morning sickness doesn't respond to the crackers and ginger ale everyone is recommending, and feels like it's more serious, push for further testing. Don't take no for an answer when your health and your hormones are at stake.

Sunny didn't give up, even though her doctor gave her every reason to.

I was 22 when I noticed I had gained 40 pounds in five months and then my period stopped. I knew I wasn't pregnant because I didn't have a boyfriend for two years, let alone the last time I had sex I was barely 19. Then it was 11 months after that I was "late" before I saw a doctor, so there was no doubt in my mind I wasn't pregnant (ha ha), but now my mind was worked up in a frenzy. What was wrong with me? Why did I feel so crappy? Was I losing my mind? How come I was always forgetting things? Did I have early dementia? I have always had my period regularly even when I was a teenager. When my doctor looked at me and said, "The reason you aren't having your period is you are *fat*," that word just rung in my ears. I felt hurt and betrayed. He also told me why I was tired—because I was *overweight* and I was *overweight* because I was tired. My face burned with shame. Then he proceeded to tell me I was *fat* because I didn't exercise. (Mind you he didn't even ask me even if I was exercising. Which I did. I swam every night for one hour, but that didn't matter to him.) I was some lumpy, dumpy, fat girl who just ate too much, didn't exercise enough and now … I was being punished for those "sins." But deep inside me I knew something wasn't right. I knew my own body and how it use to feel. But I couldn't convince this arrogant doctor there was something more than just weight.

After marrying and trying unsuccessfully to get pregnant, Sunny saw a new doctor, who "didn't make assumptions," and instead ran a battery of tests and diagnosed her hypothyroidism. According to Sunny:

> I was actually relieved to have learned of this and not have the doctors think I am some crazy fat girl anymore. I am not pregnant yet. But now I know that "yet" is a very real possiblity. I have a better relationship with my husband. I am not that cranky ol' hag anymore. But the most exciting thing is to truly feel alive again and that's a very good feeling. I am in control.

## Prepare Before Cancer Treatments

If you have cancer before you have started or completed having children, you need to have a serious sit-down discussion with the doctor before you proceed with treatment. Some cancer treatments, including radiation, chemotherapy, and surgeries, can impair fertility, or destroy eggs. It is very important that you discuss options with your doctor, such as freezing eggs and ovarian tissue, or even surgically moving ovaries away from areas to be treated so as to protect your fertility later.

## Don't Delay Childbearing

This is going to be controversial advice to some of you, but I would be overlooking an important point if I didn't say it. If you have a thyroid condition or thyroid autoimmunity and want to have children, don't delay childbearing. I'm not suggesting you run out and have children with the first guy who comes along. But so many women today feel that we have endless time to have children. Married or not, we may devote our twenties to education and our thirties to career advancement, and only take time to think about having children in our late thirties or forties. We see celebrities having babies well into their forties and even fifties, or hear about babies born to 60-year-old women, and we think we have all the time in the world.

But we don't.

Women who are having babies later in life may have an extremely good family history—for example, a mother who ovulated well into her fifties or who was able to conceive and carry a child in her forties. Celebrities may also not be telling the whole story. You rarely hear how much it cost them to have a baby using assisted reproduction technologies, or whether donor eggs or donor embryos were actually used instead of their own eggs. A child born to a late-forties celebrity may truly be a million-dollar baby.

And for every woman who conceives late in life, there are 10 more out there spending a fortune trying, women whose emotional pain and physical hardships we don't hear about because they're too disappointed to share their stories.

The reality is, fertility has a time limit for women. Even women without hormonal challenges have a sharp drop in fertility from age 35 to 40. But that drop often occurs far earlier in women with thyroid disease or thyroid autoimmunity. And thyroid disease and autoimmunity also introduce a variable into the hormonal mix, a variable that has the potential to interfere with cycles, ovulation, the ability to become pregnant, and the ability to stay pregnant even if you can conceive.

So if you are weighing your options and postponing childbearing untill your career is launched or you finances are more secure, please keep in mind that the longer you delay having a child, the greater the chance that your dream of children may never be realized.

## Don't Smoke

Smoking worsens your thyroid disease—and in some people, it's actually a trigger that brings on the thyroid condition. It can decrease your fertility. It can make you go into menopause earlier. And it shortens your lifespan and raises your risk of cancer, heart disease, stroke, and emphysema. I know—my mother died of lung cancer in her early sixties. I lost her at far too young an age. She smoked for 30 years.

But I'm also incredibly sympathetic to smokers. I was a hard-core smoker throughout my twenties. I loved smoking.

But there's a point where you simply must stop, and if you want to have a baby, you *have* to stop.

Get help wherever and however you can. Whether you need a short course of tranquilizers, the nicotine patch, Wellbutrin antidepressant, a support group, therapy, a gym membership, counseling, a 12-step program, or, like me, you drop out of society for a few weeks and crochet about seven giant afghans nonstop, find what works and stick with it to quit.

## Don't Ever Get a Hysterectomy Without a Second, a Third, or Even a Fourth Opinion

While hysterectomy is an irreversible and often life-changing surgery for women, it's viewed by many practitioners as a simple, one-size-fits-all solution to reproductive problems, from heavy periods, to pelvic pain, to difficult menopause. Since the 1960s, hysterectomy has been one of the most frequently performed inpatient surgical procedures in the United States. The prevailing attitude about hysterectomy was summed up by Dr. Ralph White, speaking at a 1971 meeting of the American College of Obstetrics and Gynecology, when he said of the

uterus: "It's a useless, bleeding, symptom-producing, potentially cancer-bearing organ."

Unfortunately, today's medical wisdom hasn't come very
far, and hysterectomy is the second most common surgery for
women in the United States, where approximately 600,000
hysterectomies are performed annually. Hysterectomy rates are
highest among younger women, age 40 to 44 years, most often
to treat fibroid tumors, endometriosis, and uterine prolapse.
More than one-fourth of American women have had hysterectomies by the time they are 60 years of age: an estimated 20
million American women. Interestingly, American women are
twice as likely to have a hysterectomy as British women and
four times more likely than Swedish women.

Many hysterectomies are unnecessary. According to a study
reported on by the American Medical Association, about 50 percent of the hysterectomies performed each year in the United
States are unnecessary. The Hysterectomy Education Resources
& Services (HERS) Foundation says the number of unnecessary
hysterectomies is far higher. According to their findings, 98 percent of women the HERS Foundation has referred to board-cer-
tified gynecologists after being told they needed hysterectomies
found that they had, in fact, not needed them.

So before you make an irreversible decision that may affect
nearly every aspect of your health and well-being, talk to a
number of experts to investigate alternatives.

## Consider Baseline and Periodic Hormonal Testing

Women who want to be in tune with their hormones may wish
to have periodic comprehensive hormonal testing: for example,
in the twenties before pregnancy, after pregnancy, late thirties,
middle forties, and periodically thereafter as well.

Before taking any sort of hormones, a woman's baseline levels should be established, with periodic evaluation afterward to gauge results of supplementation.

Some tests must be ordered by physicians: for example, glucose tolerance tests for diabetes, certain types of allergy tests, and blood tests to evalute hormone function.

You also have the option of ordering your own hormonal blood work without a doctor's prescription. This can be done through services like HealthCheckUSA. If these tests aren't covered by your medical insurance, this approach can sometimes save money, as you don't pay a doctor's markup. This is also an option if your doctor or HMO refuses to run these tests for you. This book's website has a complete listing of various self-help laboratories for serum blood testing.

Blood testing can also be done via a minimally invasive home collection technique known as a blood-spot test. No prescription or doctor's orders are required. A test kit is sent to your home, a small finger-prick of blood is applied to a card, which is then shipped back to the lab; results are sent back to you. ZRT Laboratory, for example, does blood-spot tests for the following values:

- Fasting insulin
- Follicle-stimulating hormone (FSH)
- Luteinizing hormone (LH)
- Testosterone
- Thyroid-stimulating hormone (TSH)
- Free thyroxine (FT4)
- Free triiodothyronine (FT3)
- Thyroid peroxidase antibody (TPO)
- IGF-1
- Sex hormone–binding globulin (SHBG)

Some practitioners feel that so-called normal results from blood work do not actually mean normal function. Some tests are more of a positive-negative; for example, some of the laboratories that make "rapid" or finger-prick thyroid TSH tests simply tell you if TSH is normal or out of range. This is not enough information to detect subtle changes or conditions. Serum blood tests, and even blood-spot or finger-prick tests, show you a snapshot of that level at one point in time.

Some practitioners—holistic and integrative practitioners in particular—are increasingly recommending saliva testing for evaluation of most hormones. According to naturopathic endocrinologist Dr. Michael Borkin:

> Salivary testing is the best test method because saliva contains free fractions of stress and sex hormones. Free fractions are the utilizable hormones, those that the body actually has access to. Many studies have been conducted showing the validity of assaying these steroid hormones in saliva. The usual hormone tests, conducted with blood samples, measure total hormone production, a value that includes bound (not free) hormones that are unavailable for the body's use. It is important to measure free fractions to get an accurate picture of how sex and stress hormone levels are varying by body function and activity.

Dr. Borkin also recommends salivary tests, because of the ease of multiple tests over time, such as measuring cortisol levels at four points during a 24-hour period, to evaluate cyclical response. This is in contrast to typical hormone panels, which test the levels only at the exact time of the sampling, giving a snapshot but no sense of the cycle or up and down shifts in hormones over time.

Most hormone tests can be done by saliva testing, but perhaps the most helpful saliva test is the adrenal function test, where DHEA-S is evaluated, along with four cortisol levels—morning, noon, evening, and night—to be able to monitor what stress hormones are doing over the cycle of a day. Saliva testing also makes it easier and more convenient to test for the same hormones—for example, estrogen levels—on various days of the cycle.

## Balance Should Be the Goal

Sometimes Mother Nature really does know best. There are reasons that our hormones change over time. But there are some practitioners who believe that in order to feel our best, we must all have hormone levels of a 20-year-old, whether we're 40, 60, or 80. Supplementing hormones is, therefore, considered a magic solution to a laundry list of health concerns.

Other practitioners caution us to think about this differently. According to Dr. Michael Borkin:

> The mainstream thought in the scientific and medical communities is if something is low you simply elevate it. The problem with this philosophy is that if you change something on the left then something on the right changes.

What Dr. Borkin believes is that hormones don't operate in a vacuum; they work in concert. Changes to one hormone are likely to affect the entire hormonal array so we need to address that balance to truly enjoy improved health.

Dr. Sherrill Sellman takes issue with the idea of even viewing hormones as in "decline" and prefers to describe hormones as "rebalancing and readjusting." Dr. Sellman feels that we should respect the body's wisdom, and not attempt to solve that decline and re-create youth by supplementing hormones to more youthful levels. Again, for Dr. Sellman, balance is the key.

> Perimenopause is not necessarily a time of declining estrogen levels. Rather, it's a time when the body is making an effort to stir the ovaries into action, and some women have very high levels of estrogen during this period. High estrogen levels and low progesterone production results in estrogen dominance, which is an *imbalance*. In some women, estrogen declines, but progesterone declines even more, and the main issue is still the *imbalance* of estrogen dominance. Supplementation should seek to restore the balance of the ratio, not return estrogen and progesterone levels to premenopausal levels.

While anti-aging medicine is the frontier of tomorrow's medicine, some practitioners may take it too far and go beyond the mission of avoiding degenerative, aging-related disease, instead thinking they should turn back the clock on a woman's hormones. Actress Suzanne Somers, who has been a vocal advocate for natural hormone replacement approaches, sums up this approach when she says in her book *The Sexy Years:* "I want to take the hormones I've lost in the aging process, not simply take away the symptoms."

Overall, it's a controversial issue, and you'll find practitioners with perspectives on all sides. Some experts feel that anytime you see a hormone level that is "low" it should be supplemented; some view the ratios and balance of hormones in comparison to each other as most important; and yet others feel that optimum health means restoring hormones to levels enjoyed when we were are younger.

Ultimately, only you, in conjunction with a practitioner you trust, can and should decide which approach is best for you.

## Deal with the Root Causes Before Dealing Hormone by Hormone

If there's any advice that I urge you to strongly consider, it's that this particular journey isn't going to happen with hormone-by-hormone, procedure-by-procedure solutions. Instead, hormones, which are so interrelated, pose a true holistic challenge. You need to look at the complete picture—your lifestyle, nutrition, stress levels, hormone balance, and mind-body health—to achieve a real level of health and wellness.

Conventional medicine fails to look for or treat the root causes of women's hormonal imbalances. There's no real point to looking for the reasons why a woman has irregular periods, isn't ovulating, can't get pregnant, or is having a difficult menopause, because women can be prescribed Clomid or Pergonal or Premarin, or antidepressants, sleep aids, and dozens of other drugs. While these medications may solve specific problems in the short term, they address only symptoms, not root causes. The health and hormonal imbalances underlying the symptoms usually continue on, perhaps even getting worse, and potentially causing other conditions and diseases. Some of these drugs even come with dangerous side effects and increased risks of stroke, cancer, or other serious diseases.

Dr. Michael Borkin said in an interview online:

There are increasingly severe problems if the causes of hormonal imbalance are not addressed. Even when you supplement hormones that are too low, this does not solve the original problem. Just because a level is low, it does not mean you are going to elevate that hormone if it is being converted into another hormone.

The solution? Foundational health. Dr. Sherrill Sellman recommends that a woman should always first look to a balanced, holistic, and natural approach, including diet, supplements and herbs, and lifestyle approaches, to achieve hormonal balance.

The current emphasis on bioidentical hormones is, in some ways, a massive experiment. I'd rather restore our functions so that the body can now function naturally. Oftentimes, it's not that glands aren't functioning at all, they've simply become "tone deaf." They're not responding when they're supposed to. When we look at a more holistic approach, and support brain function, ensure optimal function of the hypothalamus and pituitary, and hormone receptors, we essentially "tune up" the endocrine system.

## Don't Get Stuck in a Traffic Jam on the Money Trail

PMS, fertility, pregnancy, and menopause are a big business. And while Occam's razor charges us to choose the simpler of two equally predictive theories, many practitioners overlook basic evaluations for fundamental issues like thyroid deficiency, blood sugar irregularities, or chronic stress in favor of batteries of expensive tests and treatments, drugs, and procedures.

How else can we explain why some women don't even get a simple thyroid test before being sent off to the gynecologists, reproductive endocrinologists, or fertility clinics for batteries of expensive tests, assisted reproductive technologies, hysterectomies, or drugs?

Carrie was sent for test after test, and experienced debilitating symptoms for years.

> I went to my endocrinologist for years and could not seem to be relieved of hypothyroid symptoms. It was always thought that it may have been the wrong dose of replacement medication, but I finally had enough when the doctor told me to see a therapist and take antidepressants. I searched for a new doctor and she immediately tested for insulin resistance. Apparently a precursor to the condition for some of us is hypothyroidism. The fatigue I experienced was so debilitating, not to mention the weight gain. To make a long story short, I have my life back. Now, I have lost weight and am down from a size to 10/12 to petite 6!

Some experts believe that the overreliance on drugs, fertility treatments, and unnecessary hysterectomy is, at its core, a financial issue. Americans now spend some $220 billion a year on prescription drugs, and some of the top-selling, most profitable drugs sold in the United States are the antidepressants and sleep aids commonly prescribed to women with hormonal imbalances and "female" problems. Until recently, hormone replacement drugs like Premarin and Prempro were at the top of the most-prescribed lists. Even after the bottom dropped out of the hormone replacement market, Premarin still remains a strong-selling drug: more than 20 million prescriptions for the drug were written in 2004. The fertility industry is booming, and with one cycle of in vitro fertilization costing an average of around $8,000—almost always out of pocket and not covered by insurance—fertility is a profitable $2 billion a year business, with estimated growth of some 20 percent per year. Hysterectomies are also big business. According to the HERS Foundation, gynecologists, hospitals, and drug companies make more than $8 billion a year from hysterectomy. As Texas-based physician Steven Hotze says, "Follow the money trail. There's more money in giving a hysterectomy to treat menopausal problems, than in a therapeutic trial of thyroid hormone."

There are always situations where these tests, treatments, procedures, surgeries, and drugs are entirely appropriate solutions. But there are many times when they are not.

Besides the profit motive, it's simply the nature of conventional medicine to offer its full arsenal of tests, drugs, treatments, and surgeries, as there simply aren't other options for most conventional practitioners.

This is why you may need to turn to more alternative, holistic—and in some cases controversial—practitioners for guidance on how best to weather hormonal conditions—and, perhaps more importantly, deal with the overall imbalances and health issues that are causing them.

## Support Your Adrenal Glands

Perhaps one of the most important breakthroughs for your thyroid health, and overall hormonal health, is recognizing the critical role of stress and your adrenal glands.

According to Dr. Michael Borkin, the adrenals are at the top of the endocrine pyramid, and are almost always the first endocrine gland in the system to break down—followed by the pancreas, thyroid, ovaries, parathyroid, pineal, pituitary, and then finally, the hypothalamus, the control and master gland for the system. The more the adrenal glands are out of balance, the worse hormonal problems tend to become, until finally, almost every aspect of endocrine health and balance can be affected.

Our adrenal glands help us cope with stress, and act as physical and emotional shock absorbers for everything life throws at us. Poor nutrition, allergens, toxins, viral infection, bacterial infection, illness, injury, smoking, overstimulation with caffeine and drugs, lack of rest, chronic exhaustion, chronic emotional and mental stressors, life stressors, and other factors keep the adrenals very busy. In some of us, this ongoing siege of stress triggers a constant state of adrenal vigilance—we're in fight-or-flight mode, stuck there permanently, releasing stress hormones that flood the hormonal system downstream, harming other endocrine organs and causing a whole cascade of imbalances.

Chronic overstimulation of the adrenal system can have a number of important effects.

- To meet the increased needs for stress hormones, the body will redirect toward production of stress hormones rather than sex hormones (an adaptive mechanism that recognizes that basic survival is a higher priority than reproduction).
- Hormones like estrogen may be overproduced, resulting in imbalances, deficiencies, and excesses of hormones that impact menstrual function, fertility, menopause, and reproductive health.
- The adrenals cannot maintain a high output indefinitely, so eventually, they slow down, and with that slowdown, the rest of the endocrine system also tends to slow down. This is when thyroid function is also frequently affected.

- Eventually, the adrenals become exhausted, levels of stress hormones drop, and the body's resistance is lower. This is a period when conditions like chronic fatigue syndrome or fibromyalgia start to be seen.

The thyroid-adrenal connection is one that is often over-looked, but it is critical to overall hormonal health. According to Drs. Richard and Karilee Shames, *thyroid treatment may not even work at all unless any adrenal problems have been addressed.*

Many people with low thyroid—standard hypothyroidism—have the same immune difficulty with their adrenal gland as they do with the thyroid, an adrenal fatigue situation. You might be dealing with a combined thyroid/adrenal problem if you are a thyroid sufferer and:

- You have particularly low stamina for stress
- You have excess mood responses after eating carbs (hypoglycemia)
- You have particularly low blood pressure (momentary light-headedness upon standing up)
- You have chronic allergies
- You are feeling "tired but wired"
- You have your best energy when others are getting ready for bed
- You have poor resistance to respiratory infections
- You have cystic breasts
- You have difficulty recuperating from extra exertion or jet lag

The adrenals become even more important as women age, because after menopause, the adrenals take over a greater share of hormone production. Prior to menopause up to 30 percent of female hormones are typically produced in the adrenals, whereas after menopause, as much as half of female hormones are produced in the adrenals.

Ultimately, hormonal health for most people will depend in part on adequate support for the adrenal glands. Some general guidelines include:

- Proper nutrition, balanced blood sugar
- Restore hormones to balance wherever possible
- Minimize emotional stress by practicing stress-reduction techniques
- Eliminate toxins and heavy metals with detoxification
- Avoid and/or treat pathogens, allergens, sensitivities
- Deal with internal stress, such as inflammation and infection through an anti-inflammatory diet, candida cleansing, and other approaches
- Allow the body to repair and regenerate by getting sufficient sleep and rest

And practitioners including Drs. Sellman, Shames, and Borkin, recommend a variety of supplements to help deal with and support the adrenal glands. (Keep in mind the following is not a recommended list of everything you should take, so don't run down to the health food store! Effective treatment needs to be customized to your particular situation; some supplements are more appropriate for people with low cortisol in later-stage adrenal fatigue, while those in earlier stages may have excessively high cortisol levels.)

- Transdermal and oral hormonal supplements
- Licorice root
- Phosphatidyl choline

- Phosphatidyl serine and Siberian ginseng
- Vitamin A
- Digestive enzymes
- Probiotics
- Alpha lipoic acid
- Royal maca
- Vitamin C
- B-complex vitamins
- Magnesium
- Kelp
- Coleus forskoli
- Ashwaganda
- Schizandra
- Rhodiola
- Panax ginseng
- L-theanine

## When You Do Need Supplemental Prescription Estrogen, Consider Estriol Instead of Estradiol

There are likely some situations where a woman must have a supplemental prescription estrogen. The manufactured estrogen products are estradiol products, but many experts recommend that you instead ask for a compounded form of estriol. Some studies have shown that high levels of estriol are actually protective against breast cancer, whereas conjugated estrogens like Premarin can pose a breast cancer risk. As Dr. Sherrill Sellman notes:

> There are 10 kinds of estrogens found in Premarin. Only two are identical to human female estrogen. The other 8 are horse estrogens, obviously, not natural to a woman's body. Premarin's carcinogenicity is stated in the package insert.

There is no reason to ever take Premarin. If a woman is truly estrogen deficient, then estriol may be appropriate, as it is considered the safest of all the estrogens.

## If You Need to Balance Hormones, Consider Bioidentical Hormones

Increasingly, some hormone experts believe that bioidentical and naturally derived hormones function more effectively than synthetic hormones. By definition, bioidentical hormones need to be taken some way besides orally—as patches, gels, or transdermal creams, for example. The reason for this is that when a medicine is taken orally, it doesn't go straight to the bloodstream in its original form. Instead, it goes to the liver and is metabolized, a process that changes its structure, sometimes fairly dramatically.

One example of this is estradiol, taken orally. When it is metabolized by the liver, estradiol is converted into estrone, a different form of estrogen. Transdermal estradiol, however, goes to the bloodstream in its original form, as estradiol.

Committing to bioidentical hormones basically rules out use of some of the more easily obtained conventional drugs like Premarin, Provera, and PremPro, and switching to:

- Manufactured prescription bioidentical hormones: for example, estradiol patches, Estrasorb estrogen cream, EstroGel, or Prometrium
- Custom-compounded bioidentical hormones, available by prescription
- Naturally derived, nonprescription bioidentical hormones, available over the counter

The popular Emerita progesterone cream is one over-the-counter product that has enjoyed great success for a number of years. Sabre Sciences also produces reputable transdermal products, like BioEst Phyto-Estrogen Formula and Bio-Femme Progesterone Formula, as well as custom-manufactured over-the-counter transdermal creams that provide both hormonal and nutritional support.

There is increasing interest in studying the side effects of these very popular forms of hormone replacement. We can expect to see more studies and investigations of these hormones in the near future.

## Get Proper Nutrition and Support Digestion

Your digestion, and what you digest, are critical factors to hormonal and overall health.

Digestively, many of us are not absorbing nutrients properly, or we have pathogens such as yeast that may be interfering with our digestive capabilities, or even have progressed to a point where we have leaky gut or permeable gut, which can harm the immune system. It's critical, then, that good digestion be ensured. This may mean testing (such as a Great Smokies analysis) for intestinal and digestive problems, and addressing those sorts of issues with anything from antibiotics, to probiotic bacteria, to digestive enzyme supplementation.

Water intake is also critical. It helps with digestion, metabolism, and detoxification, among many functions.

You'll want to avoid introducing hormones, pesticides, bacteria, and pathogens in your foods. This means you'll want to try to get organic, hormone-free meats and dairy products and organic produce whenever possible. Be careful about cooking and food-handling so you can avoid food-borne diseases like *salmonella* and *yersinia,* among others.

How and when you eat is also important. Controlling blood sugar levels reduces stress on the body and promotes hormonal balance. You'll want to eat regular meals at similarly spaced intervals whenever possible. Don't go without breakfast, and don't allow yourself to become extremely hungry—this puts extra stress on your adrenals and hormonal system.

You also want to eat low-glycemically—choosing carbohydrates that do not trigger large swings in blood sugar. And balance the protein and carbohydrates in the meals you eat, to avoid large swings in blood sugar and insulin levels. Some experts recommend a two-to-one ratio of carbohydrates to protein and fat. One very specific approach to low-glycemic, ratio-balanced eating is featured in the *Zone Diet* books and cookbooks.

## Consider Other Endocrine Support If Needed

Sometimes, instead of supplementing with the sex hormones, a more effective approach is to supplement with the precursor hormones. For example, some practitioners regularly balance out sex hormone deficiencies by providing supplemental pregnenolone. Pregnenolone, made by the adrenals, serves as a precursor for production of steroid and sex hormones such as DHEA, progesterone, testosterone, the estrogens, and cortisol. Pregnenolone is known for its ability to:

- Enhance memory and learning
- Reduce the stress response and increase resistance to stress
- Help with fatigue and energy
- Help relieve PMS and menopausal symptoms

Since pregnenolone is a precursor hormone, and one that declines as we age, as pregnenolone levels decline, so do the other hormones that are downstream, so to speak. So low-dose supplementation with pregnenolone may help rebalance and reset overall hormone levels.

Practitioners may also recommend use of DHEA, another precursor hormone made by the adrenals. DHEA is converted into testosterone and estrogen. DHEA plays a role in thyroid function, by helping with the thyroid conversion of T4 to T3. DHEA can also help counteract excess cortisol and improves resistance to infection with viruses, bacteria, and toxins. DHEA also helps build muscle and decrease body fat and improves the body's response to stress.

Another area of great interest to some practitioners is the use of supplementary cortisone at very low levels, to support adrenal function and help with energy. Cortisol allows for upstream redirection of precursor hormones back to sex hormone production, can counter inflammation, and help with unresponsive thyroid treatment. In numerous journal articles and his groundbreaking 1981 book *Safe Uses of Cortisone*, Dr. William Jeffries introduced the idea of using low physiologic doses of cortisone to deal with various conditions that result from not full adrenal failure, but adrenal fatigue or hypoadrenal function. Unfortunately, many practitioners are afraid to use cortisol, because at the higher doses typically used for serious disease, this is a powerful steroid with many side effects. But, say Drs. Richard and Karilee Shames:

> Both health practitioners and the lay public have great concern about the safety of taking oral steroids. We would like to address this issue directly by making a distinction between high-dose steroid therapy and low-dose adrenal supplementation. What we are talking about is the use of small amounts

of natural adrenal hormone (hydrocortisone) to bring slightly low adrenal function up to its proper normal daily range. This is in stark contrast to the high doses of powerful synthetic adrenal hormones commonly used to treat severe health problems, or to assist in building muscles.

For hydrocortisone therapy for adrenal fatigue, you may need to consult with a more innovative or open-minded practitioner providing comprehensive thyroid and hormonal treatment.

## Consider Working with Holistic Hormone Experts

There aren't too many of them in the United States I would recommend, but ultimately, if you can, I would urge you to consider a holistic hormone expert.

You're looking for someone who will consider your health history and overall health; look for evidence of imbalances; provide nutritional, herbal, hormonal, and mind-body recommendations and advice; and look to heal fundamental problems, as well as the symptoms that represent the tip of the health iceberg.

These are practitioners who, rather than chasing symptoms, chase down the root causes of those symptoms, and attempt to treat them in a way that encourages the body to heal, restore, and replenish.

Some holistic hormone experts will have medical degrees or degrees in osteopathy, and can incorporate prescription drugs into your overall approach when necessary. Others may be naturopaths who rely on natural, nonprescription approaches and medicines; most have affiliated prescribing physicians who can work with them when necessary.

Dr. Michael Borkin is breaking ground in this area, as perhaps one of the nation's only "naturopathic endocrinologists," he has founded a unique organization, the National Center of Endocrine Education and Research (NCEER), which focuses on educating practitioners—including doctors, endocrinologists, chiropractors, naturopaths, and holistic dentists—on how to incorporate treatment of hormonal connections and the stress response into their overall practice.

I urge you to keep informed on the status of NCEER, because as more practitioners come on board after going through Dr. Borkin's training, there will be an increasing supply of them in various parts of the country available to treat us in this more comprehensive way.

Also, in this book's Resources section, I have included a listing of some practitioners I consulted for this book. These practitioners work with patients around the world, primarily through phone consultation, and are the few people I've talked to in the course of my research who seem to have a true understanding of the connection between the thyroid hormone and general health.

A word of caution: In choosing the right practitioner, be on the lookout for one-size-fits-all practitioners. These are practitioners who, to their credit, understand a genuine piece of the puzzle, such as the role of thyroid or progesterone. Unfortunately, they stop there, and don't go on to see the bigger picture—instead, turning their energies toward tireless promotion of their particular solution. You'll hear, "Everyone who is tired or overweight needs thyroid hormone," or "All postmenopausal women should have bioidentical hormone replacement," or "Progesterone is the answer for all the hormonal symptoms."

While this book has focused on and hopefully clarified the thyroid's role in hormonal imbalances, resolving a thyroid problem is ultimately not a one-stop solution for many. Typically, when there's a thyroid disorder, it's part of a bigger imbalance in hormonal health. Lasting, long-term health requires a practitioner who looks at and treats that bigger health picture.

There's the old adage that if you give a man a hammer, every problem becomes a nail. Well, if you give a doctor some insight into thyroid or progesterone, every symptom now points to a thyroid or progesterone deficiency. You may want to steer clear of practitioners who view health problems in this way, or who are onto the latest fad diagnosis or trendy hormone, and instead look for practitioners who are looking to integrate your mental and physical health, balance your hormones, and achieve true health and wellness, rather than just resolve symptoms.

## Advocate for Yourself to Be a Success Story

I can think of no better way to illustrate the benefits of being an advocate for yourself than sharing Beth's amazing success story.

Hypothyroidism runs very strongly in my family: Grandmother, mother, father, and three sisters all have been diagnosed. I also have three brothers who may or may not have issues—they haven't been tested. Since my mother and father were diagnosed six years ago, I have routinely had TSH blood tests each year. I have no idea what my levels tested at, but all along I was told I was fine. Each year my weight continued to creep up. Four years ago, my son was born. I initially lost the majority of the pregnancy weight very quickly. Then, all of a sudden, my weight started ballooning again. I started working out and dieting. No weight came off.

Then I started to notice that I felt horrible all the time, realized that I hadn't slept through the night since I was pregnant, noticed that I had absolutely no sex drive. I developed breathing problems similar to asthma, I developed heart palpitations, and my face was puffy all the time. About a year and a half ago, I went to my doctor and told her how I felt. She agreed to test my TSH levels but told me I probably just needed to lose weight for my symptoms to go away. *Duh!!!!* As if I hadn't thought of that. I informed her that I had been on the Atkins diet and was following a pretty regular exercise program—all to no avail. In fact, I was actually gaining weight. My test results came back, and once again she told me I was fine.

One morning in late June 2005, I woke up with a terrible pain in my neck. At first I thought I was developing a sore throat, but a couple of days later I realized it was my neck in my thyroid area. I went to see the same lame, condescending doctor I had seen in the past (sorry, it took me a while to learn!). She examined me, ran blood tests, and sent me for a neck X-ray. She was confident that the blood tests wouldn't reveal anything because I had been tested in March and registered a 4.5, which was normal in her opinion. Her opinion was that I had Hashimoto's thyroiditis—for once she was right—so she gave me anti-inflammatories and sent me on my way.

I went back to my office and started researching Hashimoto's thyroiditis on the Internet. That's when I stumbled across your website. That's when I realized that I was hypothyroid, and probably had been for quite some time. That's when I realized she was using the wrong reference range to evaluate my TSH levels. I went straight from work to Barnes and

Noble and bought your book, *Living Well with Hypothyroidism*. By bedtime, I had read half of it and knew my doctor had missed diagnosing me with hypothyroidism a long time ago. I realized that she must be incredibly ignorant on the subject because with my family history and the symptoms I was reporting to her, a more aware doctor would have realized I was hypothyroid long ago. I left on vacation before my test results came back. It was the worst vacation I have ever had. I felt horrible!!! I barely had the energy to do anything. All I wanted to do was stay in the hotel room and sleep. Of course, with a 4-year-old, that was not an option, so I dragged myself around feeling like I wanted to die.

When I got home, there was a message from my doctor's office letting me know that I had tested positive for hypothyroidism, that they were phoning in a prescription for 75 mcg Synthroid to my pharmacy, and that I should check back with them in eight weeks to be retested. *Huh?* By now (after reading your book, browsing your website, and through my other research) I knew there was far more to this than simply phoning in a prescription for a one-size-fits-all drug—especially when we're talking about a drug I will need to take for the rest of my life! I called the doctor's office and left a message for her. She did not even offer me the courtesy of calling me back personally. She had her assistant call me. When I asked her about the possibility of a T4-T3 combination, she told me that Synthroid was the only thyroid drug she was willing to prescribe. By now, I knew that if she was not willing to entertain any alternative, she was likely getting incentives from the drug company—or completely ignorant of the alternatives. Since I didn't want the choice of drug I would be taking for a lifetime influenced by either of these irrelevant reasons for prescribing Synthroid,

I asked that all test results pertaining to thyroid (including previous years' test results) be faxed to me immediately. It was time to shop for a new doctor. When I received my faxed test results, my suspicions regarding how long I had been suffering from hypothyroidism were confirmed. The test results coincided with when I had begun to gain weight, suffer insomnia, lost my sex drive, and all the other horrible symptoms I had been experiencing. I knew my body and how I was supposed to feel. If I'd had a doctor all along who listened to me instead of lecturing me about weight loss, I might have avoided years of declining health and quality of life.

I remembered that your website included a directory of doctors who "got it." Using that list, I selected a doctor. I left a message, was called back within a couple of hours, and had an appointment scheduled for the next day. This is the best doctor I have ever had. Our first appointment consisted of us sitting side-by-side at a desk, going over my previous test results, talking about all of my symptoms (with him stopping to explain how they are all related), and him taking copious notes. He sent me away with a saliva test kit to test TSH, free T3, free T4, thyroid antibodies, adrenal glands, testosterone, progesterone, gluten intolerance, etc. He explained that when you are dealing with hormone systems, there is very rarely just one hormone out of whack. If you look at the big picture there are usually issues with adrenal glands and the sex hormones as well.

He explained that his preference would be to put me on a T4-T3 combo from a compounding pharmacy. He was of the opinion that the dose of Synthroid prescribed by my previous doctor was way too low based on my test results. He started me off on 100 mcg T4 and 10 mcg T3. I had been taking the

Synthroid for the last week or so and still felt horrible—I just figured it was better than nothing. I immediately replaced the Synthroid with the T4-T3 combo and started feeling better within a couple of days.

Once the doctor received my saliva test results, we scheduled an appointment to discuss the outcome. As expected, my TSH levels were through the roof and free T4 and free T3 levels were seriously low. And, it was no surprise that I showed thyroid antibodies as well. The big surprises were that I had adrenal fatigue, very low progesterone levels, elevated testosterone levels, estrogen dominance, gluten intolerance, and a milk allergy I knew nothing about. We concluded that I needed to up my thyroid dosage, begin progesterone cream supplementation, an adrenal support program, and a serious detoxification plan. In addition, I began taking the supplements you specified in your book that you take daily. To address the issue of detox and weight loss, I began Ann Louise Gittleman's Fat Flush program; as well as her Fast Track Detox. The results were nothing short of amazing. I immediately began to lose weight, my puffy face vanished, my belly began to disappear, I had tons of energy, and I just felt good! The best part is her focus on fiber—which, as you know, is absolutely vital for hypothyroid patients.

After two months of following the detox program, taking T4-T3 combo replacement, progesterone replacement, and adrenal support I took the saliva test again. Today, I visited the doctor to review the results. I've lost 25 pounds (with no exercise whatsoever because of my adrenal situation), my TSH and T4 levels have entered the low end of the normal range, my T3 levels have improved, my progesterone and testosterone levels are normal, my adrenal function is somewhat better, *and* my thyroid antibodies have completely vanished. I am sleeping much better, I'm having less cramping and lighter flow during my periods, I feel the glimmer of a sex drive, I have more energy, *and I'm finally losing weight!!!*

I am so excited because I know we're on the right track and that one day I will reach the point where I recognize myself as the person I used to be.

## Moving Forward

If there's an important message I hope you take away from this book, it's this: Millions of women are needlessly suffering from hormonal health challenges; getting tested and properly treated for a thyroid condition may be the obvious—but most often overlooked—solution. *Don't be one of these women.*

Also, if you have a diagnosed thyroid problem that is being treated now, or was treated in the past, there's another important message: The thyroid is part of a carefully balanced system, and it's very easy for the hormonal balance to be thrown off. Simply because your doctor says your thyroid is "normal" now does not mean that that tiny gland—or perhaps its absence—isn't wreaking havoc on your hormonal health in many ways. Millions of women with thyroid disease are needlessly suffering from hormonal health challenges because they are not receiving optimal treatment. *Don't be one of them.*

And when it comes to our hormones, one size never fits all. Hormonal symptoms usually are a sign of an overall imbalance, and a hormonal imbalance is usually a sign of an overall health imbalance. Think of your hormones, as Dr. Michael

Borkin puts it, as "a string of Christmas lights." If one light goes out, the whole string can go dark. Our practitioners need to stop replacing each individual bulb one at a time, and start looking at the whole string!

And finally, be realistic. Maybe someday we can all have the hormonal health of a 20-year-old well into our senior years, and put off childbearing until our fifties, but today's medicine simply doesn't support that. What we do deserve is information, careful consideration from our practitioners, safe and effective relief of troublesome symptoms whenever possible, and someone who wants to understand the bigger picture so that we can live and feel well into our senior citizenhood!

Hopefully, you've found your breakthrough here in the pages of this book. May every day bring you more breakthroughs and good health.

# Charting Your Fertility and Menstrual Reproductive Cycle

One of the most important ways to understand your unique hormonal cycle, optimize fertility, identify menstrual cycle irregularities, or practice natural family planning is to chart your fertility and menstrual cycles. Charting allows you to document irregularities, understand your monthly cycles in detail, identify when and if you are ovulating, pinpoint luteal phase problems, and get a headstart in any fertility evaluation and workup.

When I decided to try to have a baby, I was nearly 35 and under treatment for Hashimoto's thyroiditis. Because of this, I was sure I was going to have difficulty conceiving. Particularly since everything I read, from books to online, tried to convince me that it was risky even to attempt a pregnancy under these conditions, I was sure I was a textbook candidate for the fertility doctors.

Several months before I was going to start trying to get pregnant, I began charting my cycle. After a few months, I knew exactly when I was ovulating. It turned out to be much easier to get pregnant than I expected, even though I have hypothyroidism. In fact, I became pregnant several months after I started trying to conceive.

*Note:* If I could do one thing to encourage women to know and understand the whole reproductive cycle, it would be to urge you to buy the book *Taking Charge of Your Fertility*, by Toni Wechsler. This book was my guide, and I referred to it again and again. I learned about how to maximize fertility and make sure my husband and I were doing everything we could to improve our chances of getting pregnant. The book is definitely a far cry from those "Now You're a Woman" pamphlets and films on menstruation in grade school. With *Taking Charge of Your Fertility*, I completely understood my monthly cycle, when my fertility level is at its highest, and how to use basal temperature and other fertility signs to chart my monthly hormonal cycle.

## Charting Basics

### Basal Body Temperature

What is basal body temperature and why is it important when you're trying to conceive? Basal body temperature (BBT) is the temperature of your body at rest, that is, your temperature when you first wake up, before undertaking any activity whatsoever. It's helpful because it can confirm ovulation and help you figure out your luteal phase. To measure this temperature, you'll need to use a special BBT thermometer—check with your local drugstore to get one. Take your temperature at the same time every morning while you are still in bed, and chart the results. Your BBT will be lower during the two weeks prior to ovulation, generally anywhere from 97.0 to 97.5 degrees Fahrenheit, as estrogen levels keep the temperature fairly low. However, right after ovulation, progesterone takes center stage and raises body temperature approximately 0.4 to 0.6 degrees until you get your next period. If you are ovulating, you'll be able to see the spike up in temperature that coincides with ovulation. Charting also lets you identify the approximate window during which you are most fertile— the best time to have intercourse if you want to get pregnant.

## Intercourse

Note that you'll also want to mark down the days when you have intercourse. There is a place on the chart I have provided to do this.

## Cervix

The cervix itself changes throughout your cycle; by monitoring it, you can also track where you are in your cycle. After your menstrual period, the cervix is dry, feels very firm and closed, and low. As you get closer to ovulation, the cervix begins to feel softer, then goes to a medium, and then high and open position right around ovulation. After ovulation, the cervix returns to the lower, closed, harder state.

## Cervical Fluid

You can also chart the course of your cycle by checking your cervical mucus, as it changes according to where you are in your cycle. Simply get a sample of your cervical fluid—you can get it from the outer edges of your vaginal opening—and stretch it between the thumb and index finger, to evaluate consistency.

*Dry:* Generally, at the start of your cycle, typically right after your period, cervical mucus is scanty and the vaginal area is dry.

*Sticky or creamy:* As the cycle progresses, the cervical mucus becomes slightly sticky or creamy. If you try to stretch the mucus between your fingers, it will break.

*Egg white:* Cervical mucus increases in volume and becomes stretchier. When you are at your most fertile, it becomes clear, very slippery, and stretchy, much like raw egg whites. This mucus is seen during the time when the chance of conception is highest.

*Watery:* After ovulation, mucus tends to become watery, and is no longer stretchy.

### Ovulation Predictor Kits

While charting allowed me to estimate ovulation, I also used an over-the-counter ovulation predictor kit, available for around $15 to $20 at the drugstore, to confirm ovulation and make sure I knew what I was doing with the charting. There are numerous kits on the market, but all of them include several reactive strips, which you urinate on. The strips work by detecting the level of luteinizing hormone (LH), a chemical that signifies oncoming ovulation, in your urine. Most kits feature blue, pink, or purple lines that become darker as ovulation draws nearer. Because these are fairly pricey, it's probably best not to use these until you have at least a ballpark estimate of when you're likely to be ovulating.

There's a place on your chart to mark results from an ovulation predictor kits.

### Ovulatory Pain

Some women can pinpoint their ovulation exactly because they feel a pain at ovulation. The pain is called mittelschmertz, German for "middle pain." Ovulatory pain can be felt in the lower abdomen, rectal area, or sometimes as a feeling of heaviness or swelling in the abdomen. The pain is due to nerve stimulation from either the increased size of the ovary or the bleeding and fluid that is released from the ruptured follicle.

### Menstrual Charting

The chart also includes space to monitor your menstrual specifics.

- Menstrual flow: heavy (a pad an hour), medium, light, or spotting
- Menstrual flow color: dark red, bright red, or brown
- Menstrual clots: large clots (bigger than a quarter), medium clots (size of a dime), or small clots (size of a raisin)

You can also chart the presence of other symptoms, such as PMS and other cyclical symptoms such as:

- Cramps
- Bloated feeling/weight gain
- Headaches
- Sore breasts
- Emotional symptoms

## Using Your Chart

With a three-month or longer history of basal temperatures and cervical changes, and with the ovulation predictor kits, you should be able to plot your cycle fairly accurately and identify your optimal fertility times. If you have been unable to get pregnant after charting and timing your intercourse during optimum fertility times, your charts will be helpful information when you go for a more thorough fertility workup with your practitioner.

Your charts are also helpful in identifying PMS symptoms and timing or in identifying cyclical irregularities.

## Fertility and Menstrual Tracking Chart

**FERTILITY & MENSTRUAL TRACKING CHART**

Name: _____  Dates covered: ____/ ____/ ____ to ____/ ____/ ____
Last 12 Cycles: Shortest _____ Longest _____ This Cycle's Length _____
Last Thyroid Test Date: _____ TSH: ____ Free T4: _____ Free T3: _____ Drug/Dose: _____

| Cycle Day | 1 | 2 | 3 | 4 | 5 | 6 | 7 | 8 | 9 | 10 | 11 | 12 | 13 | 14 | 15 | 16 | 17 | 18 | 19 | 20 | 21 | 22 | 23 | 24 | 25 | 26 | 27 | 28 | 29 | 30 | 31 |
|---|---|---|---|---|---|---|---|---|---|---|---|---|---|---|---|---|---|---|---|---|---|---|---|---|---|---|---|---|---|---|---|
| Day of week | | | | | | | | | | | | | | | | | | | | | | | | | | | | | | | |
| Date | | | | | | | | | | | | | | | | | | | | | | | | | | | | | | | |
| Time Taken | | | | | | | | | | | | | | | | | | | | | | | | | | | | | | | |
| AM Body Temp 99.1 | | | | | | | | | | | | | | | | | | | | | | | | | | | | | | | |
| 99.0 | | | | | | | | | | | | | | | | | | | | | | | | | | | | | | | |
| 98.9 | | | | | | | | | | | | | | | | | | | | | | | | | | | | | | | |
| 98.8 | | | | | | | | | | | | | | | | | | | | | | | | | | | | | | | |
| 98.7 | | | | | | | | | | | | | | | | | | | | | | | | | | | | | | | |
| 98.6 | | | | | | | | | | | | | | | | | | | | | | | | | | | | | | | |
| 98.5 | | | | | | | | | | | | | | | | | | | | | | | | | | | | | | | |
| 98.4 | | | | | | | | | | | | | | | | | | | | | | | | | | | | | | | |
| 98.3 | | | | | | | | | | | | | | | | | | | | | | | | | | | | | | | |
| 98.2 | | | | | | | | | | | | | | | | | | | | | | | | | | | | | | | |
| 98.1 | | | | | | | | | | | | | | | | | | | | | | | | | | | | | | | |
| 98.0 | | | | | | | | | | | | | | | | | | | | | | | | | | | | | | | |
| 97.9 | | | | | | | | | | | | | | | | | | | | | | | | | | | | | | | |
| 97.8 | | | | | | | | | | | | | | | | | | | | | | | | | | | | | | | |
| 97.7 | | | | | | | | | | | | | | | | | | | | | | | | | | | | | | | |
| 97.6 | | | | | | | | | | | | | | | | | | | | | | | | | | | | | | | |
| 97.5 | | | | | | | | | | | | | | | | | | | | | | | | | | | | | | | |
| 97.4 | | | | | | | | | | | | | | | | | | | | | | | | | | | | | | | |
| 97.3 | | | | | | | | | | | | | | | | | | | | | | | | | | | | | | | |
| 97.2 | | | | | | | | | | | | | | | | | | | | | | | | | | | | | | | |
| 97.1 | | | | | | | | | | | | | | | | | | | | | | | | | | | | | | | |
| 97.0 | | | | | | | | | | | | | | | | | | | | | | | | | | | | | | | |
| 96.9 | | | | | | | | | | | | | | | | | | | | | | | | | | | | | | | |
| Intercourse | | | | | | | | | | | | | | | | | | | | | | | | | | | | | | | |
| Cervix | | | | | | | | | | | | | | | | | | | | | | | | | | | | | | | |
| Cervical Fluid | | | | | | | | | | | | | | | | | | | | | | | | | | | | | | | |
| Ovulation Kit +/- | | | | | | | | | | | | | | | | | | | | | | | | | | | | | | | |
| Ovulatory Pain | | | | | | | | | | | | | | | | | | | | | | | | | | | | | | | |
| Menstrual Flow | | | | | | | | | | | | | | | | | | | | | | | | | | | | | | | |
| Menstrual Color | | | | | | | | | | | | | | | | | | | | | | | | | | | | | | | |
| Menstrual Clots | | | | | | | | | | | | | | | | | | | | | | | | | | | | | | | |
| Cramps | | | | | | | | | | | | | | | | | | | | | | | | | | | | | | | |
| Bloated/Weight | | | | | | | | | | | | | | | | | | | | | | | | | | | | | | | |
| Headaches | | | | | | | | | | | | | | | | | | | | | | | | | | | | | | | |
| Sore Breasts | | | | | | | | | | | | | | | | | | | | | | | | | | | | | | | |
| Emotional Symptoms | | | | | | | | | | | | | | | | | | | | | | | | | | | | | | | |
| Miscellaneous Notes | | | | | | | | | | | | | | | | | | | | | | | | | | | | | | | |

**KEY TO CODES USED**

| | | Flow color | DR: Dark Red \| BR: Bright Red \| B: Brown |
|---|---|---|---|
| Cervical Fluid | D: Dry \| S: Sticky \| C: Creamy \| E: Eggwhite \| W: Watery | Flow | H: Heavy \| M: Medium \| L: Light \| Sp: Spotting |
| Cervix | CH: High \| CM: Medium \| CL: Low \| CS: Soft \| CF: Firm | Clot | LC: Large \| MC: Medium \| SC: Small |

You can also download and print out full-size copies of this chart at this book's website, http://www.thyroidbreakthrough.com.

# RESOURCES

This section features a number of resources to help you obtain further information and support. Additional resources are also available at the website for this book, located at http://www. thyroidbreakthrough.com. At the site, you'll find current listings for organizations and their contact information, current website addresses, links to online sources where you can get more information about any books that are mentioned, and other helpful resources. New resources of interest to thyroid patients are also featured regularly in my patient newsletter, *Sticking Out Our Necks*.

## Mary Shomon's Health and Thyroid Information

### Websites

**Mary Shomon's "Thyroid-Info" Website**
http://www.thyroid-info.com
The Internet's most popular thyroid patient website, featuring information on all facets of thyroid disease, including both conventional and alternative approaches to diagnosis and treatment. Find chats, support groups, doctors, books, newsletters,

online forums, and more to help you in your effort to live well
with thyroid disease.

**Thyroid Top Doctors Directory**
http://www.thyroid-info.com/topdrs
A directory of patient-recommended top thyroid practitioners
from around the country and the world, organized by state and
country.

**Thyroid Site at About.com**
http://thyroid.about.com
Founded and managed by Mary J. Shomon, the thyroid site at
About.com features hundreds of articles, links to top sites on the
Internet, a weekly newsletter, support community, and more.

**Sticking Out Our Necks: The Thyroid Patient Newsletter**
*Sticking Out Our Necks* is my newsletter, designed to keep thyroid
patients up-to-date on important thyroid-related and health
news—both conventional and alternative. I scour the health
wires, medical journals, and alternative medicine sources in the
United States and around the world, looking for information
that promises better diagnosis, treatment, and symptom relief
for people with thyroid problems. Articles look at the latest information on weight loss, or up-to-the-minute news on the thyroid drugs and their manufacturers, your inspiring letters and
testimonials about the solutions you are finding that help you
live well, in-depth looks at linkages between thyroid and allergies,
thyroid and fertility, and much more. A unique feature of *Sticking Out Our Necks* is the regular reporting on new developments
in complementary and alternative medicine that have promise
in dealing with all facets of thyroid disease, as well as treatment
for unresolved thyroid symptoms. Finally, unlike other patient-

oriented newsletters, *Sticking Out Our Necks* has no affiliations with any pharmaceutical companies or patient groups. This leaves me free to be honest and up-front, telling it like it is about thyroid drugs and treatments and pharmaceutical company politics that have an impact on *your* quality of life. A paid print subscription includes a 12-page issue every other month, packed full of news and information similar to what you've found in this book, information that helps you live well. News highlights and online links are available in the free e-mail newsletter edition.

**Sticking Out Our Necks Print Newsletter**
http://www.thyroid-info.com/subscribe.htm
Write or call:
Sticking Out Our Necks/Thyroid-Info
P.O. Box 565, Kensington, MD 20895–0565
888-810-9471

**Sticking Out Our Necks E-mail Newsletter**
http://www.thyroid-info.com/newsletters.htm
A monthly e-mail newsletter, featuring summaries of key thyroid news, developments, links, interviews, and more. To subscribe, visit the website or e-mail: thyroidnews@thyroid-info.com

**Living Well with Hypothyroidism: What Your Doctor Doesn't Tell You ... That You Need to Know**
Mary J. Shomon
HarperCollins, 2005
http://www.thyroid-info.com/book.htm
This best-selling book, first published in 2000, was updated and revised in a second edition published in 2005. *Living Well with Hypothyroidism* features conventional and alternative information on every aspect of hypothyroidism, from getting diag-

nosed, to treatment, to alternatives, to residual symptoms such as fatigue and weight gain. Special issues such as pregnancy, depression, and life after thyroid cancer are explored, and a comprehensive resources section offers guidance on where to go and who to see for additional help and better health.

### Living Well with Graves' Disease and Hyperthyroidism: What Your Doctor Doesn't Tell You . . . That You Need to Know

Mary J. Shomon

HarperCollins, 2005

http://www.thyroid-info.com/graves

A comprehensive look at the conventional and alternative approaches to Graves' disease and hyperthyroidism, including the first detailed protocol for natural management of an overactive thyroid. Evaluates the pros and cons of the key treatments, including antithyroid drugs, radioactive iodine, surgery, and natural approaches. Explores nutritional approaches and long-term management of Graves' disease and hyperthyroidism.

### The Thyroid Diet: Manage Your Metabolism for Lasting Weight Loss

Mary J. Shomon

HarperCollins, 2004

http://www.GoodMetabolism.com

The first book to tackle the critical connection between weight gain and thyroid disease, offering a conventional and alternative plan for lasting weight loss. A *New York Times* and Amazon. com bestseller, a Quills Award semifinalist, the book identifies the frustrating impediments to weight loss for thyroid patients and offers solutions—both conventional and alternative—to help. With food lists, menus, supplement recommendations, handy worksheets to use in tracking weight loss and a special resource section featuring websites, books, and support groups, the book offers vital help for the millions of thyroid patients dealing with weight problems.

## Living Well with Autoimmune Disease: What Your Doctor Doesn't Tell You ... That You Need to Know

Mary J. Shomon

HarperCollins, 2002

http://www.autoimmunebook.com

After numerous printings, *Living Well with Autoimmune Disease* has established itself as the definitive guide to understanding mysterious and often difficult-to-pinpoint autoimmune disorders like thyroid disease, Hashimoto's thyroiditis, Graves' disease, multiple sclerosis, rheumatoid arthritis, Sjögren's syndrome, lupus, alopecia, irritable bowel syndrome, psoriasis, Raynaud's, and many others—and offers a road map to finding both conventional and alternative diagnosis, treatment, recovery—and in some cases, even prevention or cure! *Alternative Medicine Magazine* has said, "*Living Well with Autoimmune Disease* should not only prove inspirational for those afflicted with these mysterious conditions, but also offers solid, practical advice for getting your health back on track."

## Living Well with Chronic Fatigue Syndrome and Fibromyalgia: What Your Doctor Doesn't Tell You ... That You Need to Know

Mary J. Shomon

HarperCollins, 2004

http://www.cfsfibromyalgia.com

The book and website feature an integrative approach to diagnosis and treatment of chronic fatigue syndrome and fibromyalgia, two conditions that are more common in thyroid patients, and that share similar symptoms. While most books promote one particular theory and treatment approach, *Living Well with Chronic Fatigue Syndrome and Fibromyalgia* looks at the bigger picture, by exploring a myriad of theories and treatment options—from conventional therapies such as medication and vitamins, to alternative approaches, including yoga and massage. The book and site feature descriptions of risk factors and symptoms and a detailed checklist you can use to aid in self-evaluation and diagnosis with your physician. *Living Well with Chronic Fatigue Syndrome and Fibromyalgia* is the first book to provide a comprehensive, personalized plan for those suffering with CFS and fibromyalgia.

## Thyroid-Related Websites

### Thyroid-Info / Thyroid Information
http://www.thyroid-info.com
Home page for this book, and for my monthly news report, *Sticking Out Our Necks.* You'll find thyroid news and information, personal thyroid stories, and more. The site has hundreds of comprehensive, up-to-date links to the Web's best resources on hypothyroidism, thyroid disease, and health information.

### Thyroid Disease at About.com
http://thyroid.about.com
This is my thyroid disease website at About.com, part of the New York Times Company, where you'll find feature articles and links related to all facets of thyroid disease, my popular thyroid bulletin boards, a newsletter, and other information to support people with thyroid disease.

**Thyroid History**

http://www.thyroidhistory.net

Edna Kyrie's well-researched, comprehensive site features many articles covering thyroid disease and thyroid research, going back to the 1900s.

**Endocrineweb**

http://www.endocrineweb.com

A large site developed by doctors with more in-depth information on thyroid disease. Conventional focus but good depth of information, especially on surgery.

**Thyroid Disease Manager**

http://www.thyroidmanager.org

Full-length book offering detailed, highly conventional thyroid information with a medical tone and focus, primarily for doctors.

**John Johnson's Thyroid Website**

http://www.ithyroid.com

Home page for John Johnson, patient advocate and researcher of nutritional protocols for thyroid disease.

**Elaine Moore's Web Site**

http://www.elaine-moore.com

Home page for Elaine Moore, Graves' disease and autoimmune disease patient advocate and author of several excellent books on Graves' disease and Graves' ophthalmopathy.

**Alt.support.thyroid**

http://www.altsupportthyroid.org/

Patient-oriented information on the full range of thyroid issues.

**Jacob Teitelbaum's Site**
http://www.endfatigue.com
Discusses chronic fatigue syndrome, fibromyalgia, and the connection to thyroid problems.

**Broda Barnes Research Foundation**
http://www.brodabarnes.org
Features information on thyroid and adrenal conditions.

**Hormone Foundation**
http://www.hormone.org
Conventional overview information on thyroid and other hormone problems.

**American Thyroid Association**
http://www.thyroid.org
Conventional overview information on thyroid and other hormone problems.

## Thyroid-Related Books

There are a number of conventional thyroid books written by doctors and health writers, and frankly I'm not even going to list them here at all. I find them sometimes condescending, too similar to each other, and consistent in presenting a narrow, conventional, doctor-oriented, instead of patient-oriented, view. In addition to my own books, I recommend the following thyroid books to help in covering certain aspects of thyroid disease.

**Feeling Fat, Fuzzy or Frazzled?**
Drs. Richard and Karilee Shames
Hudson Street Press, 2005

**Overcoming Thyroid Disorders**
David Brownstein, M.D.
Medical Alternatives Press, 2002.
Good information on holistic and hormonal approaches to thyroid treatment.

**The Thyroid Solution: A Mind-Body Program for Beating Depression and Regaining Your Emotional and Physical Health**
Ridha Arem, M.D.
Ballantine Books, 2000
Strongest in its discussion of brain fog, depression, loss of libido, weight gain, anxiety, and the need for T3. Interesting information on the relationship of thyroid disease to brain chemistry and resulting depression, anxiety disorders, mood disorders, and other mental and emotional effects of hypothyroidism.

**Thyroid Balance**
Glenn Rothfeld, M.D.
Adams, 2002
Valuable book covering the various issues that cause the thyroid to go out of balance, including some alternative focus.

**Graves' Disease: A Practical Guide**
Elaine Moore and Lisa Moore
McFarland & Company, 2001
Excellent, comprehensive, and well-researched overview of Graves' disease and hyperthyroidism that offers conventional and alternative information on diagnosis and treatment.

## ThyroidPower: Ten Steps to Total Health
Richard Shames, M.D., and Karilee Halo Shames, R.N., Ph.D.
HarperCollins, 2002
Puts some basics of hypothyroidism's causes, test, diagnosis, and treatment into a 10-step program of information that can help patients get properly diagnosed and treated. Also extra focus on autoimmune disease.

## What Your Doctor May Not Tell You About Hypothyroidism
Kenneth Blanchard, M.D.
Warner Books, 2004
This interesting and helpful book is by popular Boston-area thyroid expert Kenneth Blanchard, who documents his innovative approach to treating hypothyroidism using a specific combination of T4 and T3 drugs.

## Hormones, Health, and Happiness
Steven F. Hotze
Forrest Publishing, 2005
Controversial, high-profile book that focuses on diagnosis of hormonal problems by symptoms and bioidentical hormone replacement.

## Solved: The Riddle of Illness
Stephen Langer, M.D., and James F. Scheer
McGraw-Hill, 2000
Langer, a follower of Broda Barnes's theories, has written what he calls the follow-up to Barnes's book. It looks at some nutritional and vitamin approaches for hypothyroidism. The book is at its best discussing supplements and nutritional approaches that might help hypothyroidism.

**Hypothyroidism: The Unsuspected Illness**
Broda Otto Barnes, M.D.
HarperCollins, 1982
This book, published more than 20 years ago, was written by the now-deceased Dr. Broda Barnes. It is considered the bible for alternative thyroid information and use of basal body temperature in diagnosis. The book is still in print but not likely to be stocked in bookstores. It is, however, available by special order, or at the Web's online bookstores. The book contains a fair amount of out-of-date information, but it is the first to truly acknowledge the wide-ranging impact the thyroid has on nearly every facet of health. Also, it doesn't talk down to patients or dismiss various health concerns.

**Your Guide to Metabolic Health**
Drs. Gina Honeyman-Lowe and John C. Lowe
McDowell Publishing Company, 2003
Excellent overview of hypometabolism, including hypothyroidism, and an integrative approach to help treat this multidisciplinary problem.

**Iodine: Why You Need It, Why You Can't Live Without It**
David Brownstein, M.D.
Medical Alternatives Press, 2004
Information on the role of iodine in thyroid disease and other health concerns.

**The Hormone Heresy: What Women Must Know About Their Hormones**
Dr. Sherrill Sellman
Getwell International, 2000
Helpful overview of hormones and the controversies surrounding use of estrogen.

# Thyroid Drug Manufacturers and Websites

**Tapazole, Levoxyl, Cytomel**

King Pharmaceuticals, Inc.

501 Fifth Street

Bristol, Tennessee 37620

Phone: 888-840-5370, 800-776-3637    Fax: 866-990-0545

http://www.kingpharm.com

Levoxyl: http://www.levoxyl.com, 866-LEVOXYL (538-6995)

Cytomel:  http://www.kingpharm.com/product_view.asp?id_
product = 36

Tapazole:  http://www.kingpharm.com/product_view.asp?id_
product = 47

Tapazole is the brand name for the antithyroid drug methimazole. Levoxyl is a levothyroxine product. Cytomel is liothyronine, the synthetic form of triiodothyronine (T3).

**Armour Thyroid, Thyrolar, Levothroid**

Forest Pharmaceuticals

Professional Affairs Department

13600 Shoreline Drive, St. Louis, MO 63045

Phone: 800-678-1605, ext.7301    Fax: 314-493-7457

http://www.forestpharm.com/

Armour Thyroid: http://www.armourthyroid.com

Thyrolar: http://www.thyrolar.com

Levothroid: http://www.levothroid.com

Armour Thyroid is a natural thyroid hormone replacement
product. Thyrolar is the brand name for liotrix, synthetic T4-
T3 levothyroxine-liothyronine combination drug. Levothroid
is a levothyroxine drug. (*Note*: Currently, Armour Thyroid and
Thyrolar are not readily available outside the United States. If
you are interested in these products in Canada or other countries, start by contacting the Broda Barnes Foundation.)

**Unithroid**

Lannett Pharmaceuticals

9000 State Road

Philadelphia, PA 19136

Phone: 800-325-9994, 215-333-9000

A brand of levothyroxine, originally made by Jerome Stevens Pharmaceuticals.

**Westhroid, Nature-Throid**

Western Research Laboratories

21602 North 21st Avenue

Phoenix, AZ 85027

Phone: 877-797-7997, 623-879-8537    Fax: 623-879-8683

http://www.westernresearchlaboratories.com

Nature-Throid and Westhroid are prescription desiccated thyroid drugs. Westhroid is a cornstarch-bound, natural thyroid hormone product. Nature-Throid is bound with microcrystalline cellulose, and is hypoallergenic.

**Synthroid**

Abbott Laboratories

100 Abbott Park Road

Abbott Park, IL 60064-3500

Phone: 800-255-5162

http://abbott.com or http://www.synthroid.com

Synthroid is the top-selling levothyroxine drug.

**Thyrogen**

Genzyme Therapeutics

500 Kendall Street

Cambridge, MA 02142

Phone: 800-745-4447, 617-768-9000

http://www.thyrogen.com

Thyrogen is a drug that, when used along with tests to detect recurrent or leftover thyroid cancer, can prevent the need to become hypothyroid as part of that testing.

## Organizations and Advocacy Groups: North America

**Broda Barnes Research Foundation**
P.O. Box 110098
Trumbull, CT 06611
Phone: 203-261-2101   Fax: 203-261-3017
http://www.brodabarnes.org
This organization was founded to advance the theories and approaches begun by the late Dr. Broda Barnes, including the basal metabolism test for thyroid disease and use of natural thyroid drugs. For a small fee, they'll send you a package of informational articles and materials, and information on doctors who practice using their approaches.

**American Foundation of Thyroid Patients**
P.O. Box 4914
Odessa, TX 79760
Phone: 432-694-9966
http://www.thyroidfoundation.org
A patient founded this thyroid organization, which offers a newsletter and other support.

**Thyroid Foundation of Canada/La Fondation Canadienne de la Thyroide**
797 Princess Street, Suite 304
Kingston, ON K7L 1G1

Phone: 613-544-8364, In Canada: 800-267-8822
Fax: 613-544-9731
http://www.thyroid.ca/
Canada's thyroid education–related organization for patients.

**American Autoimmune Related Diseases Association**
22100 Gratiot Avenue
E. Detroit, MI 48021
Phone: 586-776-3900
http://www.aarda.org
Information about autoimmune disorders, including Hashimoto's disease and Graves' disease. This organization provides
general information about autoimmune disorders and profiles
of specific diseases.

**Alt.support.thyroid**
http://www.altsupportthyroid.org
The Usenet bulletin board for thyroid patients.

**Thyroid Forums**
http://www.thyroid-info.com/forum
Links to support groups and forums on the Internet

## Professional Organizations

**National Center of Endocrine Education and Research
(NCEER)**
2233 Farady Avenue, Suite K
Carlsbad, CA 92008
Phone: 760-448-2757
http://www.NCEER.com

**The Thyroid Foundation of America**
One Longfellow Place, Suite 1518
Boston, MA 02114
Phone: 800-832-8321    Fax: 617-534-1515
http://www.allthyroid.org    http://www.tsh.org/
This is the main U.S. organization involved in thyroid education and outreach. Primarily run by doctors and medical interests, and funded in part by pharmaceutical companies, this organization stays fairly close to the official party line, but does offer decent conventional introductory information on thyroid disease.

**The Endocrine Society**
8401 Connecticut Avenue, Suite 900
Chevy Chase, MD 20815-6817
Phone: 301-941-0200    Fax: 301-941-0259
http://www.endo-society.org
Professional organization focusing on endocrine diseases, including thyroid disease, that primarily serves practitioners, but also provides information to thyroid patients.

**American Association of Clinical Endocrinologists**
1000 Riverside Avenue, Suite 205
Jacksonville, FL 32204
Phone: 904-353-7878    Fax: 904-353-8185
http://www.aace.com
The American Association of Clinical Endocrinologists (AACE) is a professional medical organization devoted to clinical endocrinology. At their website they sponsor an online Specialist Search Page, at http://www.aace.com/directory, which allows you to identify AACE members by geographic location, including international options. A unique feature is the ability to select

by subspecialty. Again, as a mainstream organization of endocrinologists, expect conventional approaches from these referrals.

**Hormone Foundation**
8401 Connecticut Avenue, Suite 900
Chevy Chase, MD 20815-5817
Phone: 800-HORMONE (800-467-6663)
http://www.hormone.org
Fact sheets and information about hormones and hormonal conditions, including thyroid disease.

**American Thyroid Association**
American Thyroid Association
6066 Leesburg Pike, Suite 650
Falls Church, VA 22041
Phone: 703-998-8890    Fax: 703-998-8893
Patient Information Line: 800-THYROID
http://www.thyroid.org
Professional organization for practitioners that also provides information to thyroid patients.

## Finding Thyroid and Other Doctors, Verifying Credentials

**Thyroid Top Docs Directory**
http://www.thyroid-info.com/topdrs
Mary J. Shomon's free state-by-state and international listing of top doctors for thyroid disease, founded in 1997.

**Armour Thyroid/Thyrolar**
Find a Prescribing Physician Database

http://www.armourthyroid.com/locate.html
A database of doctors who are open to prescribing Armour
and/or Thyrolar.

**American Association of Clinical Endocrinologists**
Find an Endocrinologist Database
http://www.aace.com/resources/memsearch.php
A source for conventional endocrinologists who are AACE
members.

**American Thyroid Association**
Find a Thyroid Specialist Database
http://www.thyroid.org/patients/specialists.php3
A source for conventional thyroid doctors who are AACE
members.

**Thyroid-Cancer.net**
Locate a Thyroid Cancer Specialist
http://www.thyroid-cancer.net/resources/findaspec.php3
A source for conventional thyroid cancer specialists.

**Endocrine Surgeons Membership List**
http://www.endocrinesurgeons.org/members/members.html
A source for endocrine surgeons.

**New York Thyroid Center Surgeon Referrals**
Phone: 212-305-0442    Fax: 212-305-0445
A source for finding conventional thyroid surgeons and specialists.

**HealthyNet Find a Practitioner**
http://www.healthy.net/scr/center.asp?centerid=53
Excellent resource for finding alternative, complementary, holistic, and herbal practitioners.

**American Osteopathic Association**

142 East Ontario Street

Chicago, IL 60611

Phone: 800-621-1773, 312-202-8000    Fax: 312-202-8200

http://www.aoa-net.org/

The American Osteopathic Association has state referral lists for osteopaths in all 50 states.

**American Medical Association Physician Select Program**

http://www.ama-assn.org/aps/amahg.htm

AMA's online Physician Select program allows you to browse their database for AMA member doctors, almost always conventional doctors. It lists medical school and year graduated, residency training, primary practice, secondary practice, major professional activity, and board certification for all doctors who are licensed physicians.

**Administrators in Medicine DocFinder Service**

http://www.docboard.org/docfinder.html

**American Holistic Health Association**

P.O. Box 17400

Anaheim, CA 92817-7400

Phone: 714-779-6152

http://www.ahha.org

The American Holistic Health Association offers an online referral to its members—holistic doctors.

**American Holistic Medical Association**

12101 Menaul Boulevard NE, Suite C

Albuquerque, NM 87112

Phone: 505-292-7788    Fax: 505-293-7582

http://www.holisticmedicine.org/

The American Holistic Medical Association publishes a Referral Directory of member M.D.s and D.O.s.

**Medical Board Charges or Actions**
http://www.fsmb.org/directory_smb.html
You can also find out if disciplinary action has even been taken with your doctor or if charges are pending against him or her, by calling your state medical board. A good list of all medical boards is found at the Federation of State Medical Boards on-line directory.

# Women's Health, Reproductive Health, Hormones

*Support, Information, Advocacy*

**American College of Obstetricians and Gynecologists**
409 12th Street SW
P.O. Box 96920
Washington, DC 20090-6920
Phone: 202-638-5577
http://www.acog.org

**Association of Reproductive Health Professionals**
2401 Pennsylvania Avenue NW, Suite 350
Washington, DC 20037
Phone: 202-466-3825    Fax: 202-466-3826
http://www.arhp.org/

**American Society for Reproductive Medicine**
1209 Montgomery Highway
Birmingham, AL 35216-2809

Phone: 205-978-5000    Fax: 205-978-5005
http://www.asrm.org
Formerly the American Fertility Society.

**National Women's Health Resource Center**
157 Broad Street, Suite 315
Red Bank, NJ 07701
Phone: 877-986-9472    Fax: 732-530-3347
http://www.healthywomen.org

**Black Women's Health Imperative**
600 Pennsylvania Avenue SE, Suite 310
Washington, DC 20003
Phone: 202-548-4000, 202-543-9743
http://www.blackwomenshealth.org
Formerly known as the National Black Women's Health Project.

**The Hormone Foundation**
8401 Connecticut Avenue, Suite 900
Chevy Chase, MD 20815-5817
Phone: 800-HORMONE (800-467-6663)
http://www.hormone.org

**American Medical Women's Association**
801 North Fairfax Street, Suite 400
Alexandria, VA 22314
http://www.amwa-doc.org

**American Association of Sex Educators, Counselors, and Therapists**
P.O. Box 1960
Ashland, VA 23005-1960
Phone: 804-752-0026    Fax: 804-752-0056
http://www.aasect.org

## Websites

**Women's Health at About.com**
http://womenshealth.about.com

**International Women's Health Coalition**
http:// www.iwhc.org

**John R. Lee, M.D.**
http:// www.johnleemd.com

**My Monthly Cycles**
http://www.mymonthlycycles.com

**Holistic GYN Site**
http://www.holisticgyn.com/index.html

**Women's Health Initiative/National Institutes of Health**
National Heart, Lung, and Blood Institute (NHLBI)
http:// www.nhlbi.nih.gov/whi

## Books

**The New Harvard Guide to Women's Health**
Karen J. Carlson, Stephanie A. Eisenstat, and Terra Ziporyn
Belknap Press, 2004

**Our Bodies, Ourselves: A New Edition for a New Era**
Boston Women's Health Book Collective
Touchstone, 2005

**Women's Health: Body, Mind, Spirit: An Integrated Approach to Wellness and Illness**
Marian C. Condon
Prentice Hall, 2002

**Hormone Heresy: What Women Must Know About Their Hormones**
Dr. Sherrill Sellman
Getwell International, 2000
http://www.ssellman.com

**Feeling Fat, Fuzzy or Frazzled?**
Drs. Richard and Karilee Shames
Hudson Street Press, 2005

**The Hormone Connection : Revolutionary Discoveries Linking Hormones and Women's Health Problems**
Gale Maleskey
Rodale Books, 2001

**Natural Hormone Balance for Women: Look Younger, Feel Stronger, and Live Life with Exuberance**
Uzzi Reiss and Martin Zucker
Atria, 2002

**The Hormonally Vulnerable Woman**
Geoffrey Redmond
Regan Books, 2005

# Puberty, Menstrual, and Sexual Issues

## Support and Information

**The Magic Foundation; Precocious Puberty**
Phone: 800-3 MAGIC 3 (800-362-4423)
http://www.magicfoundation.org/www/docs/146
A nonprofit organization for growth-related disorders offering
a ton of resources from info on clinical trials to scholarships to
information, education, and networking.

## Websites

**Menstruation Center at OBGyn Center Online**
http://obgyn.healthcentersonline.com/menstruation/?WT.
srch=1

**Heath 4 Her**
http://www.health4her.com

**Medline Plus: Puberty and Adolescence**
http://www.nlm.nih.gov/medlineplus/ency/article/001950.
htm
A service of the National Library of Medicine and the National Institutes of Health.

**Precocious Puberty, University of Michigan Health Systems**
http://www.med.umich.edu/1libr/yourchild/puberty.htm

**Kids Health for Parents: Precocious Puberty**
http://kidshealth.org/parent/medical/sexual/precocious.html
Sponsored by the Nemours Foundation.

**Kids Health for Parents: Delayed Puberty**

http://kidshealth.org/teen/sexual_health/changing_body/
delayed_puberty.html

Sponsored by the Nemours Foundation.

## Books

**Ready, Set, Grow! A What's Happening to My Body? Book
for Younger Girls**
Lynda Madaras and Linda Davick
Newmarket Press, 2003

**Early Puberty in Girls: The Essential Guide to Coping
with This Common Problem**
Paul Kaplowitz
Ballantine Books, 2004

**Taking Charge of Your Fertility: The Definitive Guide to
Natural Birth Control, Pregnancy Achievement, and Repro-
ductive Health**
Toni Weschler
HarperCollins, 2006

**Taking Back the Month: A Personalized Solution for Man-
aging PMS and Enhancing Your Health**
Diana Taylor
Perigee Trade, 2002

**Dr. Susan Lark's Heavy Menstrual Flow and Anemia Self-
Help Book**
Susan M. Lark, M.D.
Celestial Arts, 1996

**The PMDD Phenomenon: Breakthrough Treatments for Premenstrual Dysmorphic Disorder (PMDD) and Extreme Premenstrual Syndrome**
Diana L. Dell and Carol Svec
McGraw-Hill, 2002

**25 Natural Ways to Relieve PMS**
Nadine Taylor
McGraw-Hill, 2002

**Reclaiming Desire: 4 Keys to Finding Your Lost Libido**
Andrew Goldstein and Marianne Brandon
Rodale Books, 2004

## Pregnancy and Postpartum Issues

*Support, Information, Advocacy*

**Association of Women's Health, Obstetric and Neonatal Nursing**
http://www.awhonn.org
This is a professional organization for nurses that provides educational materials, promotes legislative programs, research, and coalition work with similar organizations. The association's activities are focused in three areas: childbearing and the newborn, women's health across the lifespan, and professional issues.

**American Pregnancy Association**
1425 Greenway Drive, Suite 440
Irving, TX 75038
Phone: 800-672-2296    Fax: 972-550-0800

http://www.americanpregnancy.org
The American Pregnancy Association is a national health organization committed to promoting reproductive and pregnancy wellness through education, research, advocacy, and
community awareness.

## Websites

**Obgyn.net Pregnancy and Birth Section**
www.obgyn.net/pb/pb.asp

**About.com Pregnancy**
http://pregnancy.about.com

## Books

**What to Expect When You're Expecting**
Heidi Murkoff
Workman, 2002

**Mayo Clinic Guide to a Healthy Pregnancy**
Mayo Clinic
HarperCollins, 2004

**The Everything Pregnancy Book: What Every Woman
Needs to Know Month-by-Month to Ensure a Worry-Free
Pregnancy**
Paula Ford-Martin
Adams Media Corporation, 2003

**Mothering Magazine's Having a Baby, Naturally: The
Mothering Magazine Guide to Pregnancy and Childbirth**
Peggy O'Mara, Wendy Ponte, and Jackie Facciolo
Atria, 2003

**The Mother of All Pregnancy Books: The Ultimate Guide to Conception, Birth, and Everything in Between**
Ann Douglas
Wiley, 2002


**This Isn't What I Expected: Overcoming Postpartum Depression**
Karen Kleiman and Valerie Raskin
Bantam, 1994


**Beyond the Blues: A Guide to Understanding and Treating Prenatal and Postpartum Depression**
Shoshana S. Bennett and Pec Indman
Moodswings, 2003


**Down Came the Rain: My Journey Through Postpartum Depression**
Brooke Shields
Hyperion, 2005


## Infertility and Miscarriage

*Support, Information, Advocacy*


**Resolve: The National Infertility Association**
7910 Woodmont Avenue, Suite 1350
Bethesda, MD 20814
Phone: 888-623-0744, 301-652-8585    Fax: 301-652-9375
http://www.resolve.org

This organization provides education, advocacy and support for men and women facing the crisis of infertility. They have a help line, medical call-in hour, physician referral service, member-to-member contact system, and family-building magazine.

**American Fertility Association**
666 Fifth Avenue, Suite 278
New York, NY 10103
Phone: 888-917-3777     Fax: 718-601-7722
http://www.theafa.org
National organization dedicated to educating, supporting, and advocating for men and women concerned with reproductive health, fertility preservation, infertility, and all forms of family building.

## Websites

**Infertility Resources for Consumers**
http://www.ihr.com/infertility/

**About Infertility**
http://www.infertility.about.com

**Fertility Awareness: Feminist Women's Health Center**
http://www.fwhc.org/birth-control/fam.htm

**InterNational Council on Infertility Information Dissemination**
http://www.inciid.org/

**Immunology and Pregnancy Loss**
http://www.inciid.org/immune.html

**Fertility Plus**
http://www.fertilityplus.org/

**Surviving Miscarriage: You Are Not Alone**
http://www.survivingmiscarriage.com

**Ivillage: Miscarriage and Pregnancy Loss**
http://parenting.ivillage.com/pregnancy/pmiscarriage/
topics/0,,4rrw,00.html

*Books*

**Taking Charge of Your Fertility: The Definitive Guide
to Natural Birth Control, Pregnancy Achievement, and
Reproductive Health**
Toni Weschler
HarperCollins, 2006

**Enhancing Fertility Naturally: Holistic Therapies for a
Successful Pregnancy**
Nicky Wesson
Healing Arts Press, 1999

**The Fertility Plan: A Holistic Program to Conceiving a
Healthy Baby**
Helen Caton
Fireside, 2000

**The Infertility Cure: The Ancient Chinese Wellness Pro-
gram for Getting Pregnant and Having Healthy Babies**
Randine Lewis
Little, Brown, 2005

**Coming to Term: Uncovering the Truth About Miscarriage**
Jon Cohen and Sandra Ann Carson
Houghton Mifflin, 2005

**Miscarriage: Why It Happens and How Best to Reduce Your Risks—A Doctor's Guide to the Facts**
Henry M. Lerner, M.D., and Alice D. Domar, M.D.
Perseus Books Group, 2003

**Trying Again: A Guide to Pregnancy After Miscarriage, Stillbirth, and Infant Loss**
Ann Douglas, John R. Sussman, and Deborah L. Davis
Taylor Trade Publishing, 2000

**Infertility Survival Handbook**
Elizabeth Swire-Falker
Riverhead, 2004

**What to Expect When You're Not Expecting: Infertility: What You Needed to Know . . . But No One Told You**
Ty Canady
iUniverse, 2003

**Six Steps to Increased Fertility: An Integrated Medical and Mind-Body Approach to Promote Conception**
Robert L. Barbieri, M.D., Alice D. Domar, Ph.D., and Kevin R. Loughlin, M.D.
Free Press, 2000

**The Everything Getting Pregnant Book: Professional, Reassuring Advice to Help You Conceive**
Robin Elise Weiss
Adams, 2004

# Breastfeeding

## Support, Information, Advocacy

**La Leche League**
1400 N. Meacham Road
Schaumburg, IL 60173–4808
Phone: 847-519-7730
http://www.lalecheleague.org/webus.html

## Websites

**Kelly Mom**
http://www.kellymom.com

**Ask Dr. Sears**
http://www.askdrsears.com

**Breastfeeding.com**
http://www.breastfeeding.com

**La Leche League**
http://www.lalecheleague.org

**Dr. Vince Ianelli's website**
http://pediatrics.about.com

**Keep Kids Healthy**
http://www.keepkidshealthy.com/breastfeeding

**Breastfeeding Online**
http://www.breastfeedingonline.com

**ProMoM: Promotion of Mother's Milk**
http://www.promom.org

**Breastfeeding Basics**
http://www.breastfeeding-basics.com/html/info.html

## Books

**The American Academy of Pediatrics New Mother's Guide to Breastfeeding**
Joan Younger Meek, ed.
Bantam, 2002

**The Breastfeeding Book: Everything You Need to Know About Nursing Your Child from Birth Through Weaning**
Martha Sears and William Sears
Little, Brown, 2000

**The Womanly Art of Breastfeeding, 7th rev. ed.**
La Leche League International
Plume

# Perimenopause and Menopause

### Support, Information, Advocacy

**North American Menopause Society**
P.O. Box 94527
Cleveland, OH 4410
Phone: 800-774-5342, 440-442-7550    Fax: 440-442-2660
Email: info@menopause.org
http://www.menopause.org

**Hysterectomy Education Resources**
**Services Foundation**
422 Bryn Mawr Avenue
Bala Cynwyd, PA 19004

Phone: 610-667-7757, 888-750-HERS (888-750-4377)
http://www.hersfoundation.com


## Websites

### Project AWARE/Menopause

http://www.project-aware.org/Experience/whatismeno.shtml

### Power Surge

http://www.power-surge.com

### Menopause Online

http://www.menopause-online.com

### Perimenopause Natural Supplement Guide

http://www.bloomingtonwebguide.com/perimeno.htm

### Mayo Clinic Information

http://www.mayoclinic.com/health/perimenopause/DS00554

### About.com Women's Health on Menopause

http://womenshealth.about.com/od/menopause/

### OBgyn.net/Menopause

http://www.obgyn.net/meno/meno.asp

### Medline Plus Menopause

http://www.nlm.nih.gov/medlineplus/menopause.html

### Menopausal Hormone Use: Questions and Answers

http://www.cancer.gov/newscenter/estrogenplus
National Cancer Institute fact sheet.

## Books

**What Your Doctor May Not Tell You About Menopause:**
**The Breakthrough Book on Natural Hormone Balance**
John R. Lee, M.D., and Virginia Hopkins
Warner Books, 2004

**What Your Doctor May Not Tell You About PREmenopause:**
**Balance Your Hormones and Your Life from Thirty to Fifty**
John R. Lee, M.D., Jesse Hanley, M.D., and Virginia Hopkins
Warner Books, 1999

**Hormone Heresy: What Women Must Know About Their**
**Hormones**
Dr. Sherrill Sellman
Getwell International, 2000

**Before the Change: Taking Charge of Your Perimenopause**
Ann Louise Gittleman
HarperSanFrancisco, 2004

**New Menopausal Years, The Wise Woman Way:**
**Alternative Approaches for Women 30–90**
Susun Weed
Ash Tree Publishing, 2001

**Could It Be…. Perimenopause? How Women 35–50 Can**
**Overcome Forgetfulness, Mood Swings, Insomnia, Weight**
**Gain, Sexual Dysfunction and Other Telltale Signs of Hor-**
**monal Imbalance**
Laurie Ashner and Steven R. Goldstein
Little, Brown, 2000

**Hormones, Health, and Happiness**
Steven F. Hotze
Forrest Publishing, 2005

**The Power of Perimenopause: A Woman's Guide to Physical and Emotional Health During the Transitional Decade**
Stephanie Bender
Three Rivers Press, 1999

**The Hormone Survival Guide for Perimenopause: Balance Your Hormones Naturally**
Nisha Jackson
Lakefield Publishing, 2004

**Dr. Susan Love's Menopause and Hormone Book: Making Informed Choices**
Susan M. Love, M.D., and Karen Lindsey
Three Rivers Press, 2003

**Users Guide to Easing Menopause Symptoms Naturally: Learn How to Prevent Hot Flashes and Other Symptoms Safely and Naturally**
Cynthia M. Watson
Basic Health Publications, 2003

**The Wisdom of Menopause**
Christiane Northrup
Bantam, 2003

**Living Well with Menopause**
Carolyn Chambers Clark
HarperCollins, 2005

## Drug Information—General

**RxList**
http://www.rxlist.com
A professional site, featuring in-depth information on various drugs.

**WebMD Drug Checker**

http://my.webmd.com/medical_information/drug_and_herb

Consumer-oriented information on drugs and herbs.

## Compounding Pharmacies

These are some compounding pharmacies that will service mail order prescriptions and have expertise in preparing thyroid drugs, including time-released T3.

**Village Green**

5415 Cedar Lane

Bethesda, MD 20814

Phone: 800-869-9159    Fax: 301-493-4671

Prescriptions: 301-530-1112

http://www.myvillagegreen.com

E-mail: info@myvillagegreen.com

**The Compounder Pharmacy**

575 W. Illinois Avenue

Aurora, IL 60506–2956

Phone: 630-859-0333    Fax: 630-859-0114

http://www.theCompounder.com

Email: info@theCompounder.com

**Knowles Apothecary**

10400 Connecticut Avenue

Kensington, MD 20895

Phone: 301-942-7979    Fax: 301-942-5542

## Herbs, Supplements, and Vitamins

**Whole World Botanicals**

P.O. Box 322074

Ft. Washington Station

New York, NY 10032
Phone: 212-781-6026, 888-757-6026
http://www.wholeworldbotanicals.com
Company that sells high-quality organic maca, and other South
American medicinal plants and herbs.

**iHerb.com**
5012 4th Street
Irwindale, CA 91706
Phone: 866-328-1171, 626-939-7800     Fax: 626-338-1326
http://www.iherb.com

## Hormonal Medicine Practitioners

**Dr. Michael Borkin**
Sabre Sciences
2233 Faraday Avenue, Suite K
Carlsbad, CA 92008
Phone: 888-285-9098, 760-448-2750     Fax: 760-448-2751
http://www.sabresciences.com

**Dr. Steven Hotze**
Hotze Health and Wellness Centers
20214 Braidwood Drive, Suite 215
Katy, TX 77450
34 South Wynden Drive, Suite 100
Houston, TX 77056
Phone: 877-577-1900, 281-579-3600
http://www.hotzehwc.com

**Sherrill Sellman, N.D.**
P.O. Box 690416
Tulsa, OK 74169-0416

Phone: 877-215-1721, 918-437-1058    Fax: 918-437-1258
http://www.ssellman.com

**Richard Shames, M.D., Karilee Shames, PhD., RN**
Phone: 707-665-0775
http://www.ThyroidPower.com
http://www.fatfuzzyfrazzled.com
E-mail: ThyroidPower@aol.com

## Hormone Testing Laboratories and Information

**Douglas Laboratories**
600 Boyce Road
Pittsburgh, PA 15205
Phone: 800-245-4440, 888-368-4522
http://www.douglaslabs.com
Sells only to licensed practitioners, but has interesting prod-
ucts, including Estro-Mend, Progesto-Mend, Testo-Quench,
Testo-Gain.

**BioHealth Diagnostics**
2929 Canon Street
San Diego, CA 92106
Phone: 800-570-2000, 619-223-7074    Fax: 800-720-7239
Consumer site: http://www.biohealthinfo.com
Practitioner site: http://www.biodia.com

**ZRT Laboratory**
1815 NW 169th Place, Suite 5050
Beaverton, OR 97006
Phone: 503-466-2445    Fax: 503 466-1636
Hormone Hotline: 503-466-9166
http://www.salivatest.com

**Diagnos-Techs, Inc.**
Clinical and Research Laboratory
6620 S. 192nd Place, Bldg. J
Kent, WA 98032
Phone: 800-878-3787
http://www.diagnostechs.com

**Great Smokies Diagnostic Laboratory/Genovations**
63 Zillicoa Street
Asheville, NC 28801
Phone: 800-522-4762, 828-253-0621
https://www.gsdl.com

# General Conventional Health Information—
## Central Websites

### WebMD

**http://my.webmd.com**
Well-organized, informative general medical site, including
conventional and some alternative information.

### About.com Health

**http://home.about.com/health**
Collection of personal expert guide–managed sites on a variety
of health topics and medical conditions.

### National Library of Medicine's PubMed

**http://www.ncbi.nhn.nih.gov/PubMed**
This is the Web's premier medical research source, offering an
easy searchable database of abstracts and journal references
from major medical journals for more than 30 years.

## Medscape

**http://www.medscape.com**
While primarily for health professionals, Medscape offers in-depth articles that explore the medical aspects of various issues, usually written in English consumers can understand.

## Intellihealth

**http://www.intellihealth.com**
High-quality, overall medical site sponsored by Johns Hopkins.

# Complementary and Alternative Medicine Resources

**American Association of Oriental Medicine**
P.O. Box 162340
Sacramento, CA 95816
Phone: 866-455-7999, 916-443-4770    Fax: 916-443-4766
http://www.aaom.org

**National Certification Commission for Acupuncture and Oriental Medicine**
11 Canal Center Plaza, Suite 300
Alexandria, VA 22314
Phone: 703-548-9004    Fax: 703-548-9079
http://www.nccaom.org

**Herb Research Foundation**
4140 15th Steet
Boulder, CO 80304
Phone: 303-449-2265    Voice mail: 800-748-2617
Fax: 303-449-7849
http://www.herbs.org

**Center for Mind/Body Medicine**
5225 Connecticut Avenue NW, Suite 414
Washington, DC 20015
Phone: 202-966-7338
http://www.cmbm.org

**American College for Advancement in Medicine**
http://www.acam.org

## Find a Holistic or Alternative Practitioner

**NCCAOM Practitioner Database**
http://dol.jkmcomm.com/acupuncture

**Acupuncture.com's Acufinder**
http://www.acufinder.com/

**Institute for Traditional Medicine Practitioner Finder**
http://www.itmonline.org/pract.htm

**HealthyNet Find a Practitioner Database**
http://www.healthy.net/scr/center.asp?centerid = 53

**American Association of Naturopathic Physicians**
http://www.naturopathic.org/

**American Osteopathic Association**
http://www.aoa-net.org/

*Websites*

**Dr. Andrew Weil**
http://www.drweil.com

**Alternative Medicine**
http://altmedicine.about.com

**Holistic Healing**
http://healing.about.com

**Spiral Visions**
http://www.spiralvisions.com

## Books

**Prescription for Nutritional Healing**
James F. Balch, M.D., and Phyllis A. Balch
Avery, 2000

**8 Weeks to Optimum Health**
Andrew Weil, M.D.
Ballantine Books, 1998

# Related Conditions and Issues

**Headaches, Migraine Disease**
http://headaches.about.com

**Mental Health Resources**
http://mentalhealth.about.com

**Heart Disease**
http://heartdisease.about.com

**Senior Health**
http://seniorhealth.about.com

**Sleep Disorders**
http://sleepdisorders.about.com

**Polycystic Ovarian Syndrome Association**
http://www.pcosupport.org

**Premature Ovarian Failure**
http://www.pofsupport.org

## Updates

Please note: If you have new resources you'd like to recommend for future updates, or if you know of updates to the information in this section, please drop me a line.
Mary J. Shomon
P.O. Box 565
Kensington, MD 20895-0565
E-mail: mshomon@thyroid-info.com

# BIBLIOGRAPHY

Alexander, EK, et al. 2004. Timing and magnitude of increases in levothyroxine requirements during pregnancy in women with hypothyroidism. *New England Journal of Medicine* 351(3):241–249.

American College of Obstetricians and Gynecologists. 2002. Thyroid disease in pregnancy. ACOG Practice Bulletin No. 37. http://www.guideline.gov/summary/summary.aspx?doc_id=3985&nbr = 003124&string = thyroid (August 2001).

Arafah, B. 2001. Increased need for thyroxine in women with hypothyroidism during estrogen therapy. *New England Journal of Medicine* 1743–1749 (August 2001).

Azizi, F. 1996. Effect of methimazole treatment of maternal thyrotoxicosis on thyroid function in breast-feeding infants. *Journal of Pediatrics* 128(6):855–858 (June 1996).

Azizi, F. 2003. Thyroid function in breast-fed infants is not affected by methimazole-induced maternal hypothyroidism: Results of a retrospective study. *Journal of Endocrinological Investigation* 26(4):301–304.

Azizi, F, et al. 2002. Thyroid function in breast-fed infants whose mothers take high doses of methimazole. *Journal of Endocrinological Investigation* 25(6):493–496 (June 2002).

Azizi, F, et al. 2003. Intellectual development and thyroid function in children who were breast-fed by thyrotoxic mothers taking methimazole. *Journal of Pediatric Endocrinology and Metabolism* 16(9):1239–1243 (December 2003).

Azizi, F, et al. 2000. Thyroid function and intellectual development of infants nursed by mothers taking methimazole. *Journal of Clinical Endocrinology and Metabolism* 85(9):3233–3238 (September 2000).

Barnard, N, et al. 2000. Diet and sex-hormone binding globulin, dys-
    menorrhea, and premenstrual symptoms. *Obstetrics and Gynecology*
    95:245–250 (2000)

Beck, GP et al. 1991. Thyroid disease and pregnancy. *Medical Clinics
    of North America* 75:121–150 (1991).

Bohles, H, et al. 1993. Development of thyroid gland volume dur-
    ing the first 3 months of life in breast-fed versus iodine-supple-
    mented and iodine-free formula-fed infants. *Clinical Investigations.*
    71(1):13–20 (January 1993).

Bohnet, HG, et al. 1981. Subclinical hypothyroidism and infertility.
    *Lancet* 2:1278 (1981).

Briggs GG, Freeman RK, and Yaffe SJ (eds). 1994. *Drugs in Pregnancy
    and Lactation,* 4th ed. Baltimore: Williams & Wilkins.

Ceccarelli, C, et al. 2001. 131I therapy for differentiated thyroid
    cancer leads to an earlier onset of menopause: Results of a ret-
    rospective study. *Journal of Clinical Endocrinology and Metabolism*
    86(8):3512–3515.

Check, JH, et al. 2005. Lymphocyte immunotherapy can improve
    pregnancy outcome following embryo transfer (ET) in patients
    failing to conceive after two previous ET. *Clinical and Experimental
    Obstetrics and Gynecology* 32(1):21–22 (2005).

Coulam, CB, et al. 1999. Immunology may be key to pregnancy loss.
    International Council on Infertility Information Dissemination.
    http://www.inciid.org.

De Groot, L, et al. (eds). Causes of hyperthyroidism. *Thyroid Disease
    Manager.* Endocrine Education, Inc. http://www.thyroidmanager.
    org/Chapter15/15–6.htm.

Doerge, DR. 2002. Goitrogenic and estrogenic activity of soy isofla-
    vones. *Environmental Health Perspectives* 110(Suppl 3):349–353 (June
    2002).

Endocrine Society, 2000. Maternal thyroid function during early
    pregnancy and neurodevelopment of the offspring. Clinical Sym-
    posium on the Impact of Maternal Thyroid Function on the Fe-
    tus and Neonate, Toronto June 21.

Phillips, NA. 2000. Female sexual dysfunction: Evaluation and
    treatment. *American Family Physician.* http://www.aafp.org/afp/
    20000701/127.html.

Fisher, D. 2005. Editorial: Next generation newborn screening for congenital hypothyroidism? *Journal of Clinical Endocrinology and Metabolism* 90(6):3797–3799.

Forrest, D. 2004. News & Views: The developing brain and maternal thyroid hormone: Finding the links. *Endocrinology* 145(9):4034–4036.

Fort, P, et al. 1990. Breast and soy-formula feedings in early infancy and the prevalence of autoimmune thyroid disease in children. *Journal of the American College of Nutrition* 9(2):164–167 (April 1990).

Freedman, R, et al. (1995). Biochemical and thermoregulatory effects of behavioral treatment for menopausal hot flashes. *Menopause: Journal of the North American Menopause Society* 2(4):211–218 (1995).

Gittleman, AL. 1998. *Before the Change: Taking Charge of Your Perimenopause.* San Francisco: HarperSanFrancisco.

Glinoer, D. 1997. The regulation of thyroid function in pregnancy: Pathways of endocrine adaptation from physiology to pathology. *Endocrine Review* 18:404.

Glinoer, D. 2003. Thyroid dysfunction in the pregnant patient. *Thyroid Manager* http://www.thyroidmanager.org/Chapter14/14-text.htm

Glinoer, D, et al. 1991. Pregnancy in patients with mild thyroid abnormalities: maternal and neonatal repercussions. *Journal of Clinical Endocrinology and Metabolism* 73:421–427.

Gotsch, G, et al. 1997. *The Womanly Art of Breastfeeding.* Judy Torgus Publisher: Plume.

Gould, D. 1998. Uterine problems: The menstrual cycle. *Nursing Standard* 12(50):38–45.

Gregoriou, G, et al. 1999. Evaluation of serum prolactin levels in patients with endometriosis and infertility. *Gynecologic and Obstetric Investigation* 48:48–51.

Haddow, JE, et al. 1999. Maternal thyroid deficiency during pregnancy and subsequent neuropsychological development of the child. *New England Journal of Medicine* 341:549–555.

Hale, TW. 2004. *Medications and Mother's Milk,* 11th ed. Amarillo, TX: Pharmasoft Publishing.

Hedrick, WR, et al. 1986. Radiation dosimetry from breast milk excretion of radioiodine and pertechnetate. *Journal of Nuclear Medicine* 27(10):1569–1571 (October 1986).

Horsby, PP, et al. 1998. Cigarette smoking and disturbance of menstrual function. *Epidemiology* 9:193–198 (1998).

Huggins, K. 1999. *The Nursing Mother's Companion.* Boston: National Book Network.

Indichova, J. n.d. An interview with Dr. Andy Silverman, Fertile Heart. http://www.fertileheart.com/articles/p.ar.silverman.html.

Indochiva, J. n.d. An interview with Shari Lieberman, Fertile Heart. http://www.fertileheart.com/articles/p.ar.shari.html.

Irvin, JH, et al. 1996. The effects of relaxation response training on menopausal symptoms. *Journal of Psychosomatic Obstetrics and Gynecology* 17(4):202–207 (1996).

Ivanhoe News Service. 2005. Sexual chemistry: Diseases and dysfunction, November. http://www.ivanhoe.com.

Jeffries, W. 1955. The present status of ACTH, cortisone, and related steroids in clinical medicine. *New England Journal of Medicine* 253:441–446 (1955).

Jeffries, W. 1967. Low dosage corticoid therapy. *Archives of Internal Medicine* 119:265–278.

Jeffries, W. 1981. *Safe Uses of Cortisol.* Springfield, IL: Charles C Thomas.

Johansen, K, et al. 1982. Excretion of methimazole in human milk. *European Journal of Clinical Pharmacology* 23(4):339–341 (October 1982).

Laumann, E, et al. 1999. Sexual Dysfunction in the United States: Prevalence and predictors. *Journal of the American Medical Association* 281:537–544. http://www.ama-assn.org/sci-pubs/journals/archive/jama/vol_281/no_6/pp0210.htm February.

Kampmann, JP. 1980. Propylthiouracil in human milk. Revision of a dogma. *Lancet* 1(8171):736–737 (April 1980).

Kaplowitz, P. 2003. Precocious puberty. *Emedicine* June 20. http://www.emedicine.com/ped/topic1882.htm.

Kennedy, RL et al. 1991. The role of hCG in regulation of the thyroid gland in normal and abnormal pregnancy. *Obstetrics and Gynecology* 78:298–307.

Krassas, GE. 2005. The male and female reproductive system in hypothyroidism. In LE Braverman et al., eds., *Werner and Ingbar's*

*The Thyroid: A Fundamental and Clinical Text*, 9th ed. Philadelphia: Lippincott Williams & Wilkins.

Krassas, GE. 2005. "The male and female reproductive system in thyrotoxicosis," in LE Braverman et al., eds., *Werner and Ingbar's The Thyroid: A Fundamental and Clinical Text*, 9th ed. Philadelphia: Lippincott Williams & Wilkins.

Langer, S. 2000. *Solved: The Riddle of Illness*, 3rd ed. New York: McGraw-Hill/Contemporary Books.

Laumann, E. et al. 1999. Sexual dysfunction in the United States: Prevalence and predictors. *Journal of the American Medical Association* 281(6):537–544.

Lawrence, R. 1999. *Breastfeeding: A Guide for the Medical Profession*, 5th ed. St. Louis: Mosby.

Lazarus, J. 2005. Sporadic and postpartum thyroiditis. In LE. Braverman et al., eds, *Werner and Ingbar's The Thyroid: A Fundamental and Clinical Text*, 9th ed. Philadelphia: Lippincott Williams & Wilkins.

Lee, A, et al. 2000. Choice of breastfeeding and physicians' advice: A cohort study of women receiving propylthiouracil. *Pediatrics* 106(1):27–30 (July 2000).

Lee, JR, et al. 2004. *What Your Doctor May Not Tell You About Menopause.* New York: Warner Books.

Lewis, R. 2004. *The Infertility Cure: The Ancient Chinese Wellness Program for Getting Pregnant and Having Healthy Babies.* Boston: Little, Brown.

Low, et al. 1979. Excretion of carbimazole and propylthiouracil in breast milk. *Lancet* 2(8150):1011.

Man, EB, et al. 1991. Maternal hypothyroidism: Psychoneurological deficits of progeny. *Annual Clinical Lab Services* 21:227–239 (1991).

Maniatis, A, et al. 2005. Congenital hypothyroidism and the 2nd newborn metabolic screen in Colorado [OR10–1]. *Endo 2005 Abstracts.*

Masuura, et al. 1990. Transient hypothyroidism in infants born to mothers with chronic thyroiditis: A nationwide study of twenty-three cases. *Endocrinology Japan* 37:369–379 (1990).

McDougall, IR, et al. 1986. Should a woman taking propylthiouracil breast-feed? *Clinical and Nuclear Medicine* 11(4):249–250.

Mestman, JH. 1997. Perinatal thyroid dysfunction: Prenatal diagnosis and treatment. *Medscape Women's Health eJournal* 2(4). www.medscape.com/viewarticle/408864.

Mohrbacher, N, et al. 2003. *The Breastfeeding Answer Book*, 3rd rev. ed. Schaurmbrug, IL: La Leche League International.

Momotani, N. 1989. Recovery from fetal hypothyroidism: Evidence for the safety of breast-feeding while taking propylthiouracil. *Clinical Endocrinology* 31(5):591–595 (November 1989).

Momotani, N. 2000. Thyroid function in wholly breast-feeding infants whose mothers take high doses of propylthiouracil. *Clinical Endocrinology* 53(2):177–181 (August 2000).

Morita, S, et al. 1998. Determining the breast-feeding interruption schedule after administration of 123I-iodide. *Annual of Nuclear Medicine* 12(5):303–306 (October 1998).

Myres, AW. 1987. Thyroid and antithyroid drugs and breast-feeding. *CMAJ* 136(9):921 (May 1987).

National Institutes of Health, National Institute of Child Health and Human Development. 2004. Do I have premature ovarian failure? U.S. Department of Health and Human Services. http://www.nichd.nih.gov/publications/pubs/pof/sub3.htm.

Nelson, L. 2005. Ovarian insufficiency. *Emedicine*, May 17. http://www.emedicine.com/med/topic3374.htm.

Newman, J, and Pitman, T. 2000. *The Ultimate Breastfeeding Book of Answers: The Most Comprehensive Problem-Solution Guide to Breastfeeding from the Foremost Expert in North America*. Roseville, CA: Prima Publishing.

Oberkotter, LV, et al. 1983. Thyroid function and human breast milk. *American Journal of Diseases of Children* 137(11):1131.

Oppenheimer, JH, et al. 1997. Molecular basis of thyroid hormone-dependent brain development. *Endocrinology Review* 18:462–475.

Prat, DE, et al. 1993. Antithyroid antibodies and the association with non-organ-specific antibodies in recurrent pregnancy loss. *American Journal of Obstetrics and Gynecology* 168(3):837–841.

Prat, DE, et al. 1993. The association of antithyroid antibodies in euthyroid nonpregnant women with recurrent first trimester abortions in the next pregnancy. *Fertility and Sterility* 60(6):1001–1005.

Readied, AM, et al. 2005. Precocious puberty with congenital hypothyroidism. *Neurology Endocrinology Letter* 26(3):253–256 (June 2005).

Rebarber, A. Antithyroid autoantibodies and recurrent pregnancy loss. Hygeia Foundation/Institute for Perinatal Loss and Bereavement. http://hygeia.org.

Riordan, J. 2004. *Breastfeeding and Human Lactation,* 3rd ed. Boston and London: Jones & Bartlett.

Robinson, PS, et al. 1994. Iodine-131 in breast milk following therapy for thyroid carcinoma. *Journal of Nuclear Medicine* 35(11):1797–1801 (November 1994).

Rothfeld, G. 2002. *Thyroid Balance: Traditional and Alternative Methods for Treating Thyroid Disorders.* Avon, MA: Adams.

Sack, J, et al. 1977. Thyroxine concentration in human milk. *Journal of Clinical Endocrinology and Metabolism* 45(1):171–173 (July 1977).

Saenz, RB. 2000. Iodine-131 elimination from breast milk: A case report. *Journal of Human Lactation* 16(1):44–46.

Scott, R Jr., et al. What Mother didn't tell you about fertility—because no one ever told her. American Fertility Association. http://www.theafa.org/faqs/afa_whatmotherdidnotsay.html.

Sellman, S. 2000. *Hormone Heresy: What Women Must Know About Their Hormones.* Tulsa: Getwell International.

Shomon, MJ. 2002. *Living Well with Autoimmune Disease: What Your Doctor Doesn't Tell You...That You Need to Know.* New York: HarperResource.

Shomon, MJ. 2004. *Living Well with Chronic Fatigue Syndrome and Fibromyalgia: What Your Doctor Doesn't Tell You ... That You Need to Know.* New York: HarperResource.

Shomon, MJ. 2005. *Living Well with Graves' Disease and Hyperthyroidism: What Your Doctor Doesn't Tell You...That You Need to Know.* New York: HarperResource.

Shomon, MJ. 2005. *Living Well with Hypothyroidism: What Your Doctor Doesn't Tell You...That You Need to Know,* 2nd ed. New York: HarperResource.

Shomon, MJ. 2004. *The Thyroid Diet: Manage Your Metabolism for Lasting Weight Loss.* New York: HarperResource.

Soldin, O. 2006. Thyroid function testing in pregnancy and thyroid disease: Trimester specific reference intervals. *Therapeutic Drug Monitor* 28(1):8–11.

Sowers, M, et al. 2003. Thyroid stimulating hormone (TSH) concentrations and menopausal status in women at the mid-life: SWAN. *Clinical Endocrinology* 58(3):340–347.

Stagnaro-Green, A, et al. 1992. A prospective study of lymphocyte-initiated immunosuppression in normal pregnancy: Evidence of a T-cell etiology for postpartum thyroid dysfunction. *Journal of Clinical Endocrinology and Metabolism* 74:645–653 (1992).

Stagnaro-Green, A, et al. 1990. Detection of at-risk pregnancy by means of highly sensitive assays for thyroid autoantibodies. *Journal of the American Medical Association* 264:1422–1425 (1990).

Van Wassenaer, AG, et al. 2002. The quantity of thyroid hormone in human milk is too low to influence plasma thyroid hormone levels in the very preterm infant. *Clinical Endocrinology* 56(5):621–627 (May 2002).

Vaquero, E, et al. 2000. Mild thyroid abnormalities and recurrent spontaneous abortion: Diagnostic and therapeutic approach. *American Journal of Reproductive Immunology* 43:204–208 (2000).

Vliet, E. 2003. *It's My Ovaries, Stupid.* New York: Scribner.

Wechsler, T. 2001. *Taking Charge of Your Fertility: The Definitive Guide to Natural Birth Control, Pregnancy Achievement, and Reproductive Health,* rev. ed. New York: HarperCollins.

Xue-Yi, C, et al. 1994. Timing of vulnerability of the brain to iodine deficiency in endemic cretinism. *New England Journal of Medicine* 221:1739–1744.

Zhang, WY, et al. 1998. Efficacy of minor analgesics in primary dysmenorrhea: A systematic review. *Journal of Obstetrics and Gynaecology* 105:780–789.

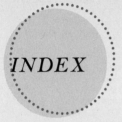

# INDEX

Page numbers in *italics* refer to figures and tables

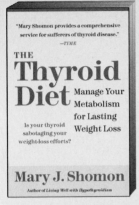
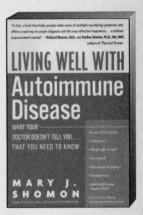
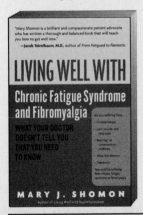